DRUGS AND THE BODY

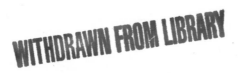

A Series of Books in Psychology

Editors:

Richard C. Atkinson
Gardner Lindzey
Richard F. Thompson

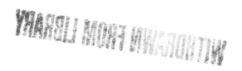

DRUGS AND THE BODY

ROBERT M. JULIEN

Department of Anesthesiology
St. Vincent Hospital and Medical Center
Portland, Oregon

W. H. FREEMAN AND COMPANY / NEW YORK

A A Z O 6 3 9

Library of Congress Cataloging-in-Publication Data

Julien, Robert M.
    Drugs and the body

    Bibliography: p.
    Includes indexes.
    1. Pharmacology.   I. Title.   [DNLM: 1. Drug Therapy.
2. Drugs—metabolism   3. Pharmacology.   QV 38 J94d]
RM300.J85 1987   615'.7   86-31873
ISBN 0-7167-1838-3
ISBN 0-7167-1842-1 (pbk.)

Printed in the United States of America

2 3 4 5 6 7 8 9 0 VB 5 4 3 2 1 0 8 9 8

To my wife, Judi
for her understanding and support

CONTENTS

In the early 1970s, while teaching and performing research in neuropharmacology, I wrote *A Primer of Drug Action*, which first appeared in 1975. In the first edition, I presented the pharmacology of psychoactive drugs so that it might be understood by readers with only modest backgrounds in biology. *A Primer of Drug Action* has been very successful; its fourth edition appeared in 1985, and it has been widely accepted by tens of thousands of students and educators in the health and social sciences.

Community interest in drug education has since broadened beyond the psychoactive drugs to drugs that affect all body systems, including prescription medications, vitamins, hormones, and poisons. Although several consumers' guides to prescription drugs are available, none present the pharmacology of these drugs in a format comprehendable to students without medical or pharmacologic backgrounds. This book attempts to fill that need.

Having extended my own education to include a medical degree, training in anesthesiology, academic teaching and research, and now community practice, I know that education is a lifelong process. Readers who have followed the evolution of the several editions of A Primer of Drug Action will see its natural progression into Drugs and the Body. I hope this current edition fulfills the needs of those who wish to extend drug education programs into more comprehensive introductions to the science of pharmacology.

I am grateful to my wife, Judi, for her selfless gift of time such that this might be written. I thank my two sons, Rob and Scott, for their help in the technical preparation of the manuscript. I also thank John Elder of Creighton University and Fred Cowan of the Oregon Health Sciences University for their review of the manuscript. Without all such help, this text would never have progressed from dream to reality.

Robert M. Julien, M.D., Ph.D.
January, 1987

INTRODUCTION

Drugs and the Body provides an introduction to pharmacology for students who want to know about certain types of drugs: those that primarily act on areas outside the brain and those that are used clinically to treat non–brain-related disorders. The material in this book builds upon material developed in *A Primer of Drug Action*; indeed, this book may be considered as a companion volume to the first when a broad scope of pharmacology is needed.

One should note, however, that this book is complete. It may be used alone by those people little concerned with the pharmacology of psychoactive drugs or those using other books of psychopharmacology or drug abuse. References to *A Primer of Drug Action* are few in *Drugs and the Body*; material from the earlier volume is not repeated here. In the present volume, I discuss most major classes of nonpsychoactive drugs, and organize the sections into autonomic pharmacology, drugs that affect the cardiovascular system, kidney, lungs, and gastrointestinal tract, hormones and vitamins, chemotherapy, immune system, and poisons. Commonly administered dosages of drugs have been omitted on purpose. Dosage always must be individualized; such medical decisions should be made only by a prescribing professional. Such information, however, is readily available in the *Physicians' Desk Reference* (PDR), published yearly by Medical Economics Company, Inc., Oradell, NJ, and in the several consumers' guides to prescription drugs. Most, but not all, available drugs or classes of drugs are included in either this book or *A Primer of Drug Action*. Once the student has mastered the information contained in these two books, he or she can readily refer to more inclusive and extensive books of pharmacology.

PHARMACOLOGY OF THE
AUTONOMIC NERVOUS SYSTEM

CHAPTER 1

INTRODUCTION TO THE AUTONOMIC NERVOUS SYSTEM

The nervous system traditionally is divided into two parts: the central nervous system and the peripheral nervous system (Figure 1.1). The central nervous system (CNS) consists of all neurons located in both the brain and the spinal cord, and the peripheral nervous system (PNS) consists of all the motor and sensory nerves situated between the CNS and the muscles, body viscera, and sense organs.

The PNS can be subdivided into afferent and efferent divisions, with the latter being further subdivided into the motor (somatic) nervous system and the autonomic nervous system. The motor component of the efferent division of the PNS innervates the skeletal

FIGURE 1.1
Major subdivisions of the nervous system. Divisions of the peripheral nervous system appear shaded.

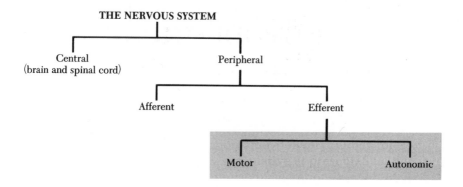

muscles, or those parts of the body that are under voluntary control, primarily the muscles of locomotion and posture. The autonomic nervous system (ANS), in contrast, supplies all of the structures of the body except the skeletal muscles. The ANS frequently is called the "visceral" nervous system since it regulates the body's functions and maintains the homeostasis of the internal organs. It does not require conscious activation and is considered to be "automatic" in its operation; it is not subject to the brain's conscious control, except through special training in such techniques as meditation or biofeedback. The ANS controls the function of the heart, the flow of blood, and the functioning of the digestive tract, and it regulates other internal functions of the body that are essential for maintaining the balance necessary for life (Levine, 1983, pp. 383–384).

Note that although the nervous system is divided into central and peripheral components, this is not a precise division. For example, the functioning of the ANS depends to some degree upon structures within the brain (such as the hypothalamus) that regulate visceral functions involving body temperature, water and electrolyte balance, body metabolism, and so on. Such division, however, allows for a clearer presentation of pharmacology.

The drugs presented in Chapters 2 and 3 (autonomic nervous system drugs) act primarily on the autonomic neurons. In order to understand the actions of these drugs, one should understand the anatomy and the physiology of the ANS.

ANATOMY AND PHYSIOLOGY OF THE AUTONOMIC NERVOUS SYSTEM

The ANS is divided into two major subdivisions, the *sympathetic* and the *parasympathetic* (Figure 1.2). Each system consists of two neurons, the preganglionic and the postganglionic. The *preganglionic* neuron has its origin within the brain stem or spinal cord, and each synapses with one or more *postganglionic* neurons, the cells bodies of which are located in specialized structures called *autonomic ganglia* (Figure 1.3). Thus, the preganglionic fibers arise from cell bodies in the spinal cord or brain stem and synapse on the postganglionic neurons, which gives rise to postganglionic fibers that innervate virtually all the internal organs except skeletal muscle.

Clinically, acetylcholine (ACh) is the neurotransmitter released by all the preganglionic neurons and by the postganglionic neurons of the parasympathetic division. The neurotransmitter released by the postganglionic neurons of the sympathetic division is norepinephrine (NE). The terms *cholinergic* and *adrenergic* describe those neurons that liberate ACh and NE, respectively. Thus, all preganglionic neurons and the postganglionic *parasympathetic* neurons are cholinergic, while postganglionic *sympathetic* neurons are most often adrenergic.

The adrenal medullae, part of the adrenal glands located on top of each kidney, present a special situation. These structures are

FIGURE 1.2
Expansion of Figure 1.1 to show two divisions of the autonomic nervous system.

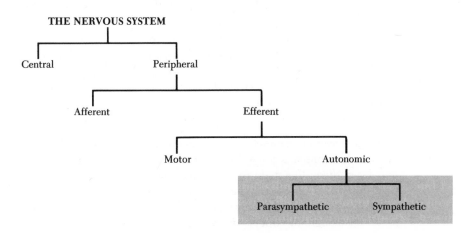

FIGURE 1.3
Sympathetic and parasympathetic divisions of the efferent limb of the autonomic nervous system. (See text for details.)

PARASYMPATHETIC OUTFLOW

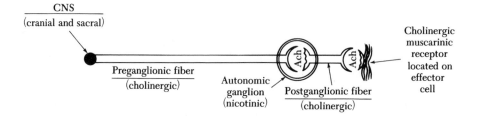

SYMPATHETIC OUTFLOW

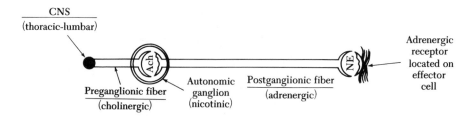

homologous to a collection of cell bodies of postganglionic sympathetic neurons. Though innervated by preganglionic (cholinergic) fibers, the cells of the adrenal medullae secrete mainly epinephrine (adrenalin) but also small amounts of norepinephrine.

Anatomically and physiologically, the preganglionic neurons of the *sympathetic* division of the ANS originate in the thoracic and lumbar segments of the spinal cord. Upon leaving the spinal cord they synapse with the postganglionic neurons, the cell bodies of which are located in clusters (*ganglia*) just alongside the spine on each side of the spinal column (Table 1.1). These clusters of postganglionic sympathetic neurons are called autonomic ganglia.

As stated by Levine:

> The paravertebral ganglia are connected to each other by nerve trunks; preganglionic fibers issuing from one level may pass up or down the chain before synapsing, or may synapse with more than one sympathetic ganglion en route. Thus a single preganglionic fiber may make contact with a large number of postganglionic fibers, and one ganglion may be inner-

TABLE 1.1
Characteristic differences between the sympathetic and parasympathetic nervous systems

	Sympathetic	Parasympathetic
Origin of preganglionic fibers	Thoracic and upper lumbar segments of spinal cord	Brainstem and sacral segment of spinal cord
Ganglia	Near CNS	Near effector cell
Length of fibers Preganglionic Postganglionic	Short Long	Long Short
Ratio of preganglionic to postganglionic fibers	High, may be 1:20 or more	Usually low—1:1 or 1:2
Response to stimulation	Diffuse	Discrete
Preganglionic transmitter	Acetylcholine (ACh)	ACh
Postganglionic transmitter	Norepinephrine (most cases)	ACh

SOURCE: R. R. Levine, *Pharmacology: Drug Actions and Reactions*, Little, Brown, Boston, 1983, p. 386.

vated by several preganglionic fibers. These ramifications of preganglionic and postganglionic fibers account in large part for the diffuse response that usually follows stimulation of the sympathetic division of the ANS (Levine, 1983, p. 386).

In the *parasympathetic* division, preganglionic neurons originate in the brain stem and the sacral segments of the spinal cord. Upon leaving the spinal cord they synapse with postganglionic neurons that cluster to form small ganglia located near the target organ that they innervate. This provides a more discrete innervation than is achieved in the sympathetic division in which postganglionic axons travel a considerable distance to the target organ.

Again, as stated by Levine:

This anatomic arrangement . . . largely accounts for the limited and discrete response that is characteristically evoked by stimulation of parasympathetic fibers (Levine, 1983, p. 386).

To understand the actions of autonomic drugs that mimic or antagonize the function of cholinergic or adenergic neurons, one should first understand the normal response of the various internal organs to autonomic nerve impulses. Most organs are supplied with postganglionic fibers arising from both divisions (Figure 1.4). The parasympathetic and sympathetic divisions, however, can be viewed as antagonistic to each other—one system augments organ

FIGURE 1.4
Autonomic innervation of various organs. (From A. Goth, *Medical Pharmacology,* 11th ed., Mosby, St. Louis, 1984.)

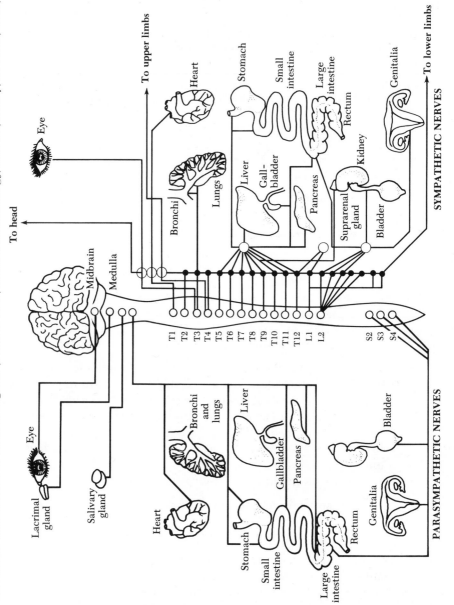

function, the other reduces it. In the heart, for example, adrenergic stimulation increases heart rate and augments the force of contraction of the heart muscle. Cholinergic stimulation slows heart rate and decreases cardiac contractility. Table 1.2 lists the responses of selected body organs to sympathetic and parasympathetic stimulation. Note from Table 1.2 and from Figure 1.5 that the receptors upon which cholinergic neurons synapse are called either *nicotinic* or *muscarinic*, and those upon which adrenergic neurons synapse are termed *alpha, beta,* and *dopaminergic*, with each of the three being subdivided into two or more subtypes. Only the beta receptors will be subdivided in this presentation.

TABLE 1.2
Responses of body organs to autonomic nerve impulses

| Effector organ | Adrenergic stimulation | | Cholinergic stimulation |
	Receptor type	Response	Response
Eye: iris, radial muscle, ciliary muscle	Alpha Beta	Mydriasis (dilated) Relaxation for far vision	Miosis (constricted) Contraction for near vision
Heart	Beta$_1$	Increased heart rate Increased contractility and conduction velocity	Decreased heart rate Decreased contractility and conduction velocity
Blood vessels Skin Skeletal muscle Abdominal viscera	Alpha Beta$_2$ Alpha	Constriction Dilatation Constriction	Dilatation
Lung Bronchial muscle	Beta$_2$	Relaxation	Contraction
Gastrointestine Motility and tone Sphincters	Beta$_2$ Alpha	Decrease Contraction	Increase Relaxation
Bladder Muscle Sphincter	Beta$_2$ Alpha	Relaxation Contraction	Contraction Relaxation
Uterus	Beta$_2$	Relaxation	
Sex organs, male	Alpha	Ejaculation	Erection
Skin (sweat glands)			Secretion
Fat cells	Beta$_1$	Lipolysis	
Salivary glands		Thick mucus	Watery saliva

SOURCE: Adapted from R. M. Julien, *Understanding Anesthesia*, Addison-Wesley, Palo Alto, CA, 1984.

FIGURE 1.5
Expansion of Figure 1.2 to show receptor types of efferent nerves on the peripheral nervous system. Receptor subdivisions for alpha and dopaminergic receptors are not included.

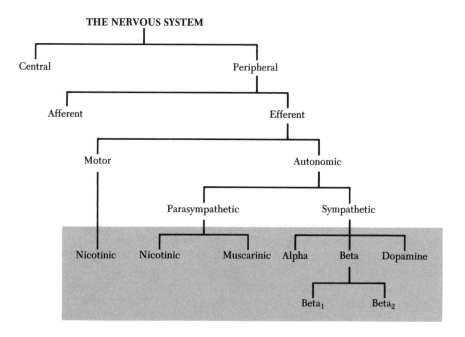

The sympathetic and parasympathetic divisions serve different functional roles in homeostasis. The parasympathetic nervous system is concerned primarily with conserving and restoring energy. It decreases heart rate, lowers blood pressure, constricts the pupil of the eye (thus protecting it from excessive light), increases contractility of the intestine and urinary bladder to aid in their emptying, and aids in the digestion and absorption of food and nutrients.

The sympathetic nervous system, on the other hand, protects the individual from environmental change and provides the rapid response necessary for coping with emergencies and stress-related situations. Discharge of the sympathetic nervous system leads to increases in heart rate, blood pressure, blood sugar, blood flow to skeletal muscles, and respiratory rate, and a reduction in blood flow to the stomach and intestinal tract. All these actions prepare the individual for handling stress. The release of adrenalin and norepinephrine from the adrenal medulla also contributes to this response.

In Chapters 2 and 3, we will see how various groups of drugs affect the functioning of the autonomic nervous system.

READINGS

Appenzeller, O., *The Autonomic Nervous System*. Elsevier, Amsterdam, 1982.

Cooper, J. R., F. E. Bloom, and R. H. Roth, *The Biochemical Basis of Neuropharmacology*, 4th ed., Oxford University Press, New York, 1982.

Goth, A. (ed.), *Medical Pharmacology*, 11th ed., Mosby, St. Louis, 1984.

Levine, R. R., *Pharmacology: Drug Actions and Reactions*, 3d ed., Little, Brown, Boston, 1983.

Weiner, N., and P. Taylor, "Neurohumoral Transmission: The Autonomic and Somatic Motor Nervous Systems," in A. G. Gilman, L. S. Goodman, T. W. Rall, and F. Murad (eds.), *The Pharmacological Basis of Therapeutics*, Macmillan, New York, 1985, pp. 66–99.

CHAPTER 2

DRUG ACTION AT ADRENERGIC NERVE TERMINALS

Norepinephrine (NE) is a neurotransmitter released by most post-ganglionic neurons of the sympathetic division of the ANS. Neurotransmitters released from the adrenal medulla include epinephrine (Epi, adrenalin) and small amounts of NE. All receptors activated by either Epi or NE are called *adrenergic.*

Adrenergic stimulants include a large number of compounds that act either directly or indirectly to stimulate both alpha-adrenergic and beta-adrenergic receptors. Those acting indirectly release catecholamines from adrenergic nerve endings. Since the action of both directly and indirectly acting drugs is to mimic the action of the body's normal adrenergic transmitters, these compounds are often referred to as *sympathomimetic drugs.*

Sympathomimetic drugs include three naturally occuring neurotransmitters, two structurally similar synthetic compounds, and several nonstructurally similar drugs that mimic the actions of the naturally occurring substances. The three naturally occurring neurotransmitters are NE, Epi, and dopamine; the two structural related, synthetically produced sympathomimetics are dobutamine and isoproterenol (Figure 2.1). Collectively, these five compounds are called *catecholamines.* The structurally dissimilar sympathomimetics either directly stimulate alpha or beta receptors or release endogenous stores of Epi or NE. The noncatecholamine sympathomimetic compounds, which are listed in Table 2.1, include

---

FIGURE 2.1
Chemical structures of natural and synthetic catecholamine sympathominetics.

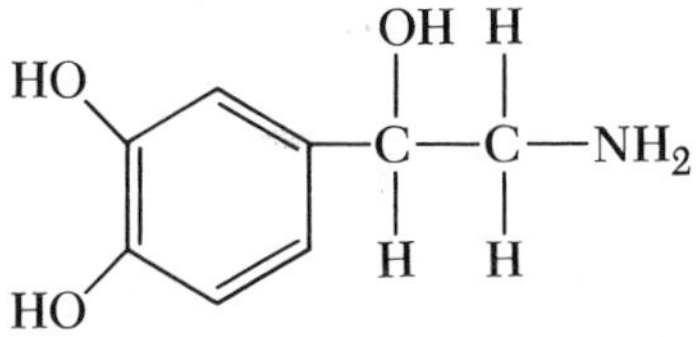

Norepinephrine

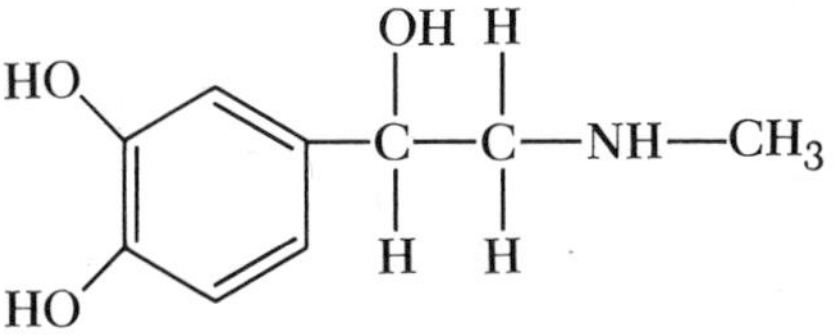

Epinephrine

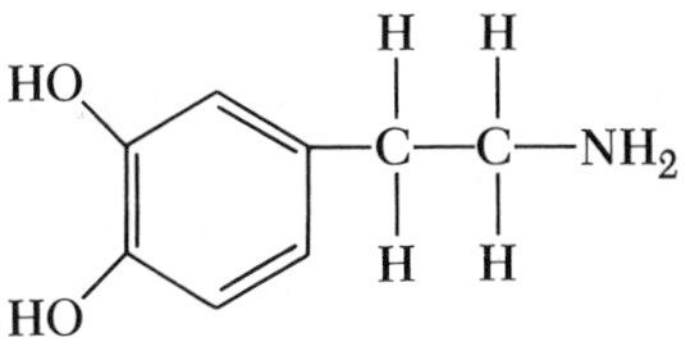

Dopamine
(Inotropin)

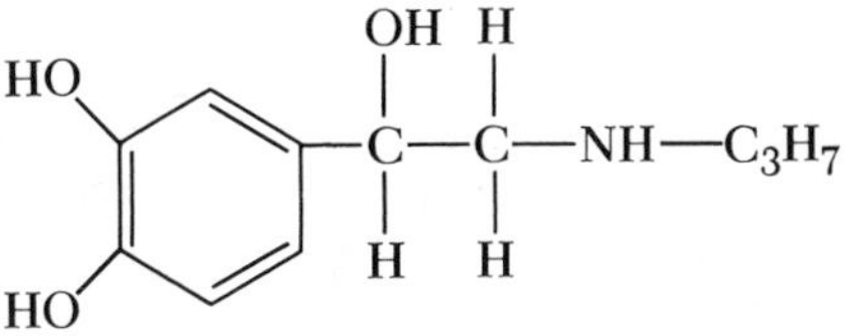

Isoproterenol
(Isuprel)

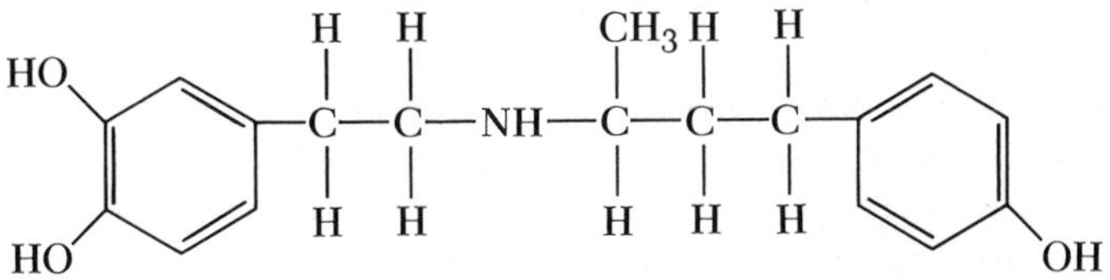

Dobutamine
(Dobutrex)

TABLE 2.1
Receptor targets and pharmacologic effects of noncatecholamine adrenergic stimulants

Drug	Receptor Alpa	Receptor Beta$_1$	Receptor Beta$_2$	Action	Clinical uses
Ephedrine	+	+ +	+ +	Directly stimulates receptor, releases NE (weak)	Vasoconstriction, bronchodilation, CNS stimulation
Mephentermine (Wyamine)	+ +	+	+	Directly stimulates receptor, releases NE	Vasoconstriction
Metaraminol (Aramine)	+ + +	+	+	Directly stimulates receptor, releases NE	Vasoconstriction
Phenylephrine (Neosynephrine)	+ + +	0	0	Directly stimulates receptor	Vasoconstriction
Methoxamine (Vasoxyl)	+ + +	0	0	Directly stimulates receptor	Vasoconstriction
Amphetamines	+ + +	+ + +	+ + +	Releases NE, directly stimulates receptor (weak)	CNS stimulation
Imipramine (Tofranil)	+ +	+	+	Blocks NE resorption	CNS stimulation
Cocaine	+ +	+	+	Blocks NE resorption	Vasoconstriction, CNS stimulation
Terbutaline (Brethine)	0	0	+ + +	Directly stimulates receptor	Bronchodilation
Isoetharine (in Bronkosol)	0	0	+ + +	Directly stimulates receptor	Bronchodilation
Metaproterenol (Alupent)	0	0	+ + +	Directly stimulates receptor	Bronchodilation
Ritodrine (Yutopar)	0	0, +	+ + +	Directly stimulates receptor	Uterine relaxation

ephedrine, several compounds that produce vasoconstriction (increase the tone and reduce the diameter of blood vessels), bronchodilators, CNS stimulants, and appetite suppressants.

The effects of these drugs on the ANS can be demonstrated from a knowledge of both the specific adrenergic receptors with which they interact, and the direct or indirect nature of their action. As Table 2.1 demonstrates, these drugs stimulate to various degrees any or all of the alpha, beta$_1$, or beta$_2$ receptors.

CATECHOLAMINE STIMULANTS

NOREPINEPHRINE

Norepinephrine, the transmitter released from most adrenergic nerve endings (postganglionic sympathetic nerves), primarily stimulates alpha receptors and only mildly stimulates beta₁ receptors. Table 2.2 lists the consequences of such alpha-receptor stimulation.

When administered intravenously at a very slow rate, NE stimulates the alpha receptors located on blood vessels of the abdominal viscera and the skin. Such stimulation results in vasoconstriction, an effect that produces a marked increase in blood pressure as a result of an increase in the resistance (or tone) of the blood vessels. While blood *pressure* is increased, however, blood *flow* to abdominal viscera (including the kidneys) is reduced. The increase in blood pressure also stimulates certain pressure receptors which, in turn, by reflex slow the heart rate and may potentially reduce car-

TABLE 2.2
Relative effects of natural and synthetic catecholamines on mean arterial pressure (MAP), heart rate (HR), cardiac output (CO), total peripheral resistance (TPR), and renal blood flow (RBF)

Drug	Receptor	Effect				
		MAP	HR	CO	TPR	RBF
Dopamine (DA)	DA (low doses)	0	0	0	0	↑↑
	DA and beta₁ (moderate doses)	↑	↑↑	↑↑↑	0	↑↑↑
	DA, beta₁, alpha (high doses)	↑↑	↑↑	↑↑	↑↑	↑↓
Norepinephrine	Alpha, mild effect on beta	↑↑↑	0, ↓	0, ↓	↑↑↑	↓↓↓
Epinephrine	Alpha, beta₁, beta₂	↑↑	↑↑	↑↑	↑	↓↓
Isoproterenol*	Beta₁, beta₂	↓	↑↑↑	↑↑↑	↓↓	↓
Dobutamine*	Beta₁	↑, 0	↑, 0	↑↑↑	↑, 0	↑, 0

* Synthetic catecholamines.
Key: ↑, 0 or ↓, 0 = little or no change.
    ↑ or ↓ = slight increase of slight decrease.
    ↑↑ or ↓↓ = moderate increase or moderate decrease.
    ↑↑↑ or ↓↓↓ = marked increase or marked decrease.
SOURCE: R. M. Julien, *Understanding Anesthesia*, Addison-Wesley, Palo Alto, CA, 1984.

diac output. Because NE produces such a large increase in peripheral vascular resistance, its ability to increase blood pressure is offset by reduced blood flow to internal organs, by increased cardiac workload since the heart must pump into a higher resistance system, and by decreased perfusion of body viscera. As a result, NE is only rarely used as the sole agent to restore blood pressure in a hypotensive patient. Its deleterious effects on perfusion and cardiac work offset the restoration of blood pressure. Other agents (discussed next) are physiologically superior to NE in restoring both blood pressure and organ perfusion.

EPINEPHRINE

Epinephrine is a direct stimulant of virtually all adrenergic receptors, including alpha, beta$_1$, and beta$_2$ receptors. It therefore produces a dose-dependent increase in both heart rate and the force of contraction (contractility), and improves cardiac output (Table 2.2). By constricting blood vessels, Epi reduces the blood flow to some vascular beds and dilates blood vessels in others, such as in skeletal muscle. Such varying actions on blood vessels supplying the viscera and skeletal muscles tend to offset each other for the most part, and the increase in the total peripheral vascular resistance, therefore, is somewhat less than one might predict. Increases in blood pressure occurring after an Epi infusion are due to cardiac stimulation rather than increased vascular resistance. Blood flow to the kidneys tends to fall as a result of vasoconstriction, but most likely it does not fall to the same extent as it does after intravenous infusion of norepinephrine.

Epinephrine's ability to dilate or relax the smooth muscle of the bronchi of the lungs can be lifesaving in disease states such as bronchial asthma. Clinically, Epi is used primarily to relieve acute attacks of asthma (bronchospasm). Because it provides local vasoconstriction, it is also used to prolong the action of local anesthetics. By constricting blood vessels in the area of injection, Epi prevents the local anesthetic from being carried away too quickly. Epi also is used to produce vigorous stimulation of the heart during such emergencies as a cardiac arrest.

DOPAMINE

Dopamine (DA) is the immediate precursor of NE. It is also a neurotransmitter in the central nervous system, where it is widely distributed. The blockade of DA receptors in the CNS is responsible for the antipsychotic and antinauseant effects of the phenothiazines and butyrophenones. Inadequate levels of DA in the CNS, specifically in the basal ganglia, on the other hand, is connected to the pathogenesis of Parkinson's disease; replacement of DA in Parkinsonian patients results in control of many of the symptoms.

In addition to its CNS neurotransmitter role, DA is a powerful cardiac stimulant. Its effect is mediated through $beta_1$ receptors on the heart, augmentation of which increases both contractility and heart rate. DA also stimulates specific DA receptors located on the renal arteries, which supply blood to the kidneys. Such stimulation produces vasodilatation of these vessels and increases blood flow to the kidneys. Because of its ability to increase both cardiac output, as a result of increased contractility and heart rate, and renal blood flow, DA is used primarily to treat certain types of shock.

ISOPROTERENOL

Isoproterenol is a synthetic catecholamine that directly stimulates $beta_1$ and $beta_2$ receptors. As a result, isoproterenol is a potent relaxant of bronchial smooth muscle and a powerful cardiac stimulant. Because it also dilates certain blood vessels, particularly those supplying the skeletal muscles, an intravenous infusion of isoproterenol increases both heart rate and cardiac contractility and, within limits, cardiac output. Because isoproterenol decreases peripheral vascular resistance, due to the vascular dilatation in skeletal muscle, its ability to increase blood pressure is limited.

Two important clinical uses follow from these effects on the lungs and the heart. Isoproterenol is widely used in the treatment of acute attacks of asthma, though such use is accompanied by marked increases in heart rate. Such an effect may reduce coronary blood flow and produce ischemia of the heart, especially in patients with coronary artery disease. Isoproterenol is also useful as a potent cardiac stimulant in patients with heart failure who do not respond to dopamine and who are able to tolerate the increased heart rate.

NONCATECHOLAMINE ADRENERGIC STIMULANTS

Several drugs that are not classified as catecholamines because of structural differences nevertheless mimic the activity of adrenergic transmitters. Some of these directly stimulate adrenergic receptors, and several indirectly increase adrenergic function by, for example, releasing NE from presynaptic nerve terminals. Table 2.1 lists several of these drugs, the receptor types upon which they work, their primary actions, and their clinical uses.

EPHEDRINE

Ephedrine is an adrenergic stimulant that both releases NE and directly stimulates alpha, beta₁, and beta₂ receptors. It is widely used as a vasoconstrictor and a bronchodilator. In the past, it has also been used as a CNS stimulant. Its effects resemble those of Epi (discussed above) but last about 10 times longer. Four drugs listed in Table 2.1 (mephentermine, metaraminol, phenylephrine, and methoxamine) stimulate alpha receptors and produce peripheral vasoconstriction. These drugs, therefore, are used to maintain adequate blood pressure when hypotension is due to vasodilatation, an uncommon occurrence. They are also widely used in nasal sprays to constrict blood vessels in the nose, thus increasing the flow of air though the nostrils. A variety of vasoconstrictors are present in numerous nasal sprays—all of these agents pharmacologically resemble these four.

As shown in Table 2.1, amphetamines are indirectly acting stimulants of alpha, beta₁, and beta₂ receptors; they exert their effect primarily by inducing the release of NE from presynaptic nerve terminals. Imipramine and cocaine are also indirectly acting sympathetic stimulants, exerting their effects by blocking the re-uptake of neurotransmitter into presynaptic nerve terminals (Julien, 1985; Cooper et al., 1982).

Three drugs listed in Table 2.1, terbutaline, isoetharine, and metaproterenol, are direct stimulants of beta₂ receptors, which makes them particularly useful in the treatment of asthma (Chapter 12). Ritodrine, also a beta₂ stimulant, is used to retard or stop premature labor in obstetrical patients because of its relaxant effects induced by beta₂ stimulation on the uterus.

ADRENERGIC BLOCKING AGENTS

Hyperactivity of the sympathetic nervous system can have deleterious effects on cardiovascular function, especially in individuals with hypertension or coronary artery disease. Many agents can reduce such excessive sympathetic activity through a variety of mechanisms (see Table 2.3), all of which result in inhibition of the actions of NE and Epi on their specific receptors. Those which primarily block adrenergic *alpha* receptors are called alpha-adrenergic blocking agents. Such an action results in vasodilatation of blood vessels, the tone of which is maintained by alpha-adrenergic activity.

Agents such as phentolamine, tolazoline, phenoxybenzamine, and prazosin are representative blockers of alpha receptors, relaxing the smooth muscle of arteries and reducing peripheral vascular resistance. These drugs occasionally are used in the treatment of peripheral vascular diseases in which spasm of the blood vessels, with reduced blood flow to the tissues, is an important clinical feature. Some of these agents also are used to manage a disease called pheochromocytoma, a tumor of the adrenal medulla characterized by excessive release of Epi and NE. These drugs block the stimulant effects of excessive levels of catecholamine on alpha receptors.

Adrenergic blocking agents that primarily block *beta* receptors are called beta-adrenergic blocking agents. (An additional subclassification currently is made to include some degree of specificity for $beta_1$ and $beta_2$ receptor blocking activity.) Dose-dependent specificity for blocking $beta_1$ receptors (primarily in the heart) aids in avoiding the bronchoconstriction that could arise from blockade of $beta_2$ receptors in the lungs. Representative beta blocking agents include propranolol, labetalol, metoprolol, nadolol, atenolol, and timolol. Of these, metoprolol and atenolol have some selectivity for blocking $beta_1$ receptors; the other three agents demonstrate less selectivity, blocking both $beta_1$ and $beta_2$ receptors.

These beta blocking drugs are used therapeutically to decrease cardiac output, heart rate, and cardiac contractility, thereby contributing to the control of hypertension, angina pectoris, and certain cardiac arrhythmias. At present, propranolol and labetalol are the only beta-adrenergic blocking agents that are available in injectable form in the United States. Neither of these are cardioselective for $beta_1$ receptors, and, in fact, labetalol is also an alpha-receptor blocker. Signs of either bronchoconstriction or excessive cardiac depression limit the use of all of these drugs. The effects of beta blocking drugs in the control of hypertension, angina, and asthma will be discussed at appropriate points later in this book.

Several other adrenergic blocking agents require brief comment. Clonidine and methyldopa affect certain specialized alpha receptors within the CNS and reduce the outflow of nerve impulses that regulate blood vessel tone. These agents are used in the treatment of hypertension, and clonidine also has proved beneficial in ameliorating some of the signs and symptoms of narcotic withdrawal in opiate addicts.

TABLE 2.3
Mechanism of action and clinical uses of adrenergic blocking agents

Drug	Mechanism of action	Clinical use
Phentolamine (Regitine)	Alpha-receptor blockade	Control of hypertension, acute and chronic
Tolazoline (Priscoline)	Alpha-receptor blockade	Control of hypertension, acute and chronic
Phenoxybenzamine (Dibenzyline)	Alpha-receptor blockade	Control of hypertension, acute and chronic
Prazosin (Minipress)	Alpha-receptor blockade	Control of hypertension, acute and chronic
Propranolol (Inderal)	$Beta_1$- and $beta_2$-receptor blockade	Control of hypertension Control of angina pectoris Control of arrhythmias, acute and chronic
Metoprolol (Lopressor)	$Beta_1$-, mild $beta_2$-receptor blockade	Control of hypertension Control of angina pectoris Control of arrhythmias, acute and chronic
Atenolol (Tenormin)	$Beta_1$-, mild $beta_2$-receptor blockade	Control of hypertension, angina, and arrhythmias (chronic)
Nadolol (Corgard)	$Beta_1$- and $beta_2$-receptor blockade	Control of hypertension, angina, and arrhythmias (chronic)
Timolol (Timoptic)	$Beta_1$- and $beta_2$-receptor blockade	Treatment of glaucoma
Labetolol (Normodyne)	$Beta_1$-, $beta_2$-, and alpha-receptor blockade	Control of hypertension, acute and chronic
Clonidine (Catapres)	Reduced central sympathetic outflow	Control of chronic hypertension
Methyldopa (Aldomet)	Reduced central sympathetic outflow	Control of chronic hypertension
Guanethidine (Ismelin)	Adrenergic neuron blocker	Control of chronic hypertension
Reserpine (Serpasil)	Adrenergic transmitter depletion	Control of hypertension Control of psychosis, acute and chronic
Methyl-tyrosine (Demser)	Inhibition of catecholamine synthesis	Control of hypertension Control of pheochromocytoma

SOURCE: Modifed from R. M. Julien, *Understanding Anesthesia*, Addison-Wesley, Palo Alto, CA, 1984.

Guanethidine and reserpine act on adrenergic nerve terminals to deplete them of transmitters. Though both drugs are used to control hypertension, they have many side effects associated with a generalized reduction in sympathetic activity.

Methyltyrosine inhibits the synthesis of adrenergic transmitters and depletes the body of its stores of Epi and NE. The drug is used only in certain particular situations, such as the preoperative preparation of patients about to undergo surgery for removal of a pheochromocytoma.

READINGS

Caritis, S. H., "Treatment of Preterm Labor: A Review of Therapeutic Options," *Drugs*, **26**:243–261 (1983).

Charney, D. S., et al., "Clonidine and Naltrexone. A Safe, Effective and Rapid Treatment of Abrupt Withdrawal from Methadone Therapy," *Arch. Gen. Psychiatry*, **39**:1327–1333 (1982).

Frishman, W. H., "Drug Therapy: Atenolol and Timolol, Two New Systemic Beta-Adrenergic Antagonists," *New Engl. J. Med.*, **306**:1456–1462 (1982).

Julien, R. M., *A Primer of Drug Action*, 4th ed., W. H. Freeman, New York, 1985.

Shand, D. G., "Drug Therapy: Propranolol," *New Engl. J. Med.*, **293**:280–284 (1975).

Souney, P. F., A. F. Kaul, and R. Osathanondh, "Pharmacology of Preterm Labor," *Clin. Pharm.*, **2**:29–44 (1983).

Weiner, N., "Norepinephrine, Epinephrine, and the Sympathomimetic Amines. Drugs that Inhibit Adrenergic Nerves and Block Adrenergic Receptors," in A. G. Gilman, L. S. Goodman, T. W. Rall, and F. Murad (eds.), *The Pharmacological Basis of Therapeutics*, 7th ed., Macmillan, New York, 1985, pp. 145–214.

Zaimis, E., "Vasopressor Drugs and Catecholamines," *Anesthesiology*, **29**:732–762 (1968).

CHAPTER 3

DRUG ACTION AT CHOLINERGIC NERVE TERMINALS

As stated in Chapter 1, acetylcholine (ACh) is the neurotransmitter liberated at the neuromuscular junction by both the pre- and the postganglionic parasympathetic neurons of the ANS and by the preganglionic neurons of the adrenergic division of the ANS. In addition, as was illustrated in Figure 1.5, the receptors activated by ACh are classified as either nicotinic or muscarinic. Nicotinic receptors are so named because the drug nicotine (in cigarettes) stimulates the autonomic ganglia and the neuromuscular junction. Muscarine, on the other hand, is a drug that preferentially stimulates acetylcholine receptors innervated by postganglionic cholinergic neurons. Based on the preferential actions of nicotine and muscarine, therefore, these two distinct types of ACh receptors in the autonomic nervous system have been characterized.

CHOLINERGIC STIMULANTS

Drugs that activate or stimulate the normal receptors for ACh are called either cholinergic stimulants or cholinomimetic drugs, since they mimic the action of acetylcholine, the normal transmitter. The various cholinergic stimulants can be divided into two major groups (Figure 3.1)—directly acting agents and inhibitors of the enzyme acetylcholinesterase. The directly acting agents may be further subdivided into (1) *nicotinic stimulants* that affect ACh receptors in autonomic ganglia and skeletal muscle and (2) *muscarinic stimulants* that affect receptors located on effector organs innervated by postganglionic cholinergic neurons. The acetylcholinesterase (AChE) inhibitors may be subdivided into (1) those that are reversible in their actions and (2) those that are irreversible.

NICOTINIC STIMULANTS

A drug classified as a nicotinic stimulant mimics the actions of ACh either at the autonomic ganglia or the neuromuscular junction. Ganglionic stimulant drugs currently have little clinical use, although they are of laboratory and historical importance. Nicotine is the classic ganglionic stimulant, although it is not used clinically. Ganglionic stimulation by nicotine results in increased heart rate and blood pressure and vasoconstriction. Smoking nicotine results in increased gastrointestinal tone and motor activity of the bowel.

FIGURE 3.1
Classification of cholinergic stimulants.

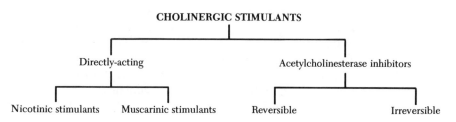

Nausea, vomiting, and diarrhea may all follow use of nicotine. Stimulation of the neuromuscular junction, however, is achieved only with quite high doses of nicotine.

MUSCARINIC STIMULANTS

Drugs that stimulate muscarinic receptors in the parasympathetic nervous system have important uses in medicine. Although their duration of action is longer, these drugs exhibit many of the actions of ACh on smooth muscles without significantly affecting autonomic ganglia or the neuromuscular junction. Despite some major limitations, these drugs have important uses in disorders of the eye, gastrointestinal tract, and urinary bladder. Since they constrict the bronchi, they should not be used in patients with a history of asthma, and because of their stimulant effects, they are probably best avoided in patients with a history of peptic ulcer. Because such drugs may predispose patients to cardiac arrhythmias by decreasing heart rate and force of contraction and altering electrical conduction, they are seldom given to patients with a history of hyperthyroidism or coronary artery disease.

Muscarinic stimulants include pilocarpine, bethanechol, and carbachol (Figure 3.2). Pilocarpine, a natural alkaloid derived from a South American shrub, produces pinpoint pupils (miosis) when the alkaloid is applied directly to the eye. Because this effect tends to lower intraocular pressure, pilocarpine is widely used as an ophthalmic solution to treat glaucoma. Bethanechol (Urecholine) is used primarily to relieve postoperative distension of the gastrointestinal tract, to increase gastrointestinal motility, and to relieve urinary retention. These uses are due to the fact that muscarinic stimulation increases the tone of the gastrointestinal tract and the bladder. Carbachol is used most frequently as an ophthalmic solution to produce postoperative miosis after intraocular surgery and to treat glaucoma.

REVERSIBLE AChE INHIBITORS

The enzyme acetylcholinesterase (AChE) is necessary to terminate the action of ACh after its release from presynaptic nerve terminals. Drug-induced inhibition of AChE leads to prolongation of the neurotransmitter action of ACh and results in longer receptor stimulation. The prototype "reversible" AChE agent is physostigmine (Eserine), an alkaloid obtained from the Calabar (or ordeal) bean (Figure 3.3). As a result of AChE inhibition, ACh levels rise and

FIGURE 3.2
Structures of acetylcholine, pilocarpine (a natural cholinomimetic alkaloid), and
two synthetic cholinomimetics.

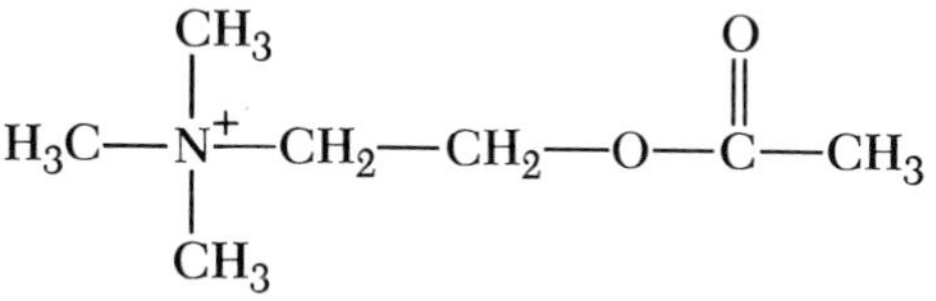

Acetylcholine

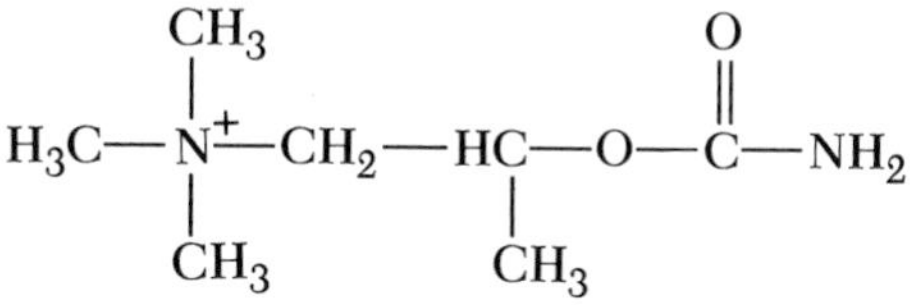

Bethanechol

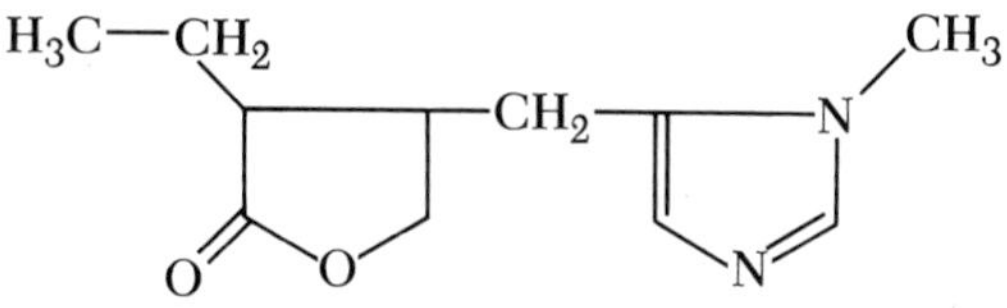

Pilocarpine

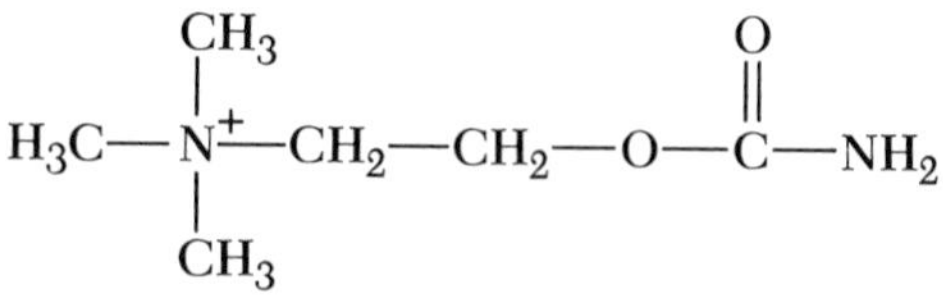

Carbachol

both muscarinic and nicotinic stimulation occur. Clinical interest
in these agents centers on the eye, the intestine, and the neuromuscular junction. When applied locally to the eye, physostigmine
causes miosis, alters the ability to focus vision, and causes intraocular pressure to fall. Though the drug may be used in the treatment of glaucoma, both the directly acting muscarinic agents discussed above and the topically applied, long-acting irreversible
AChE inhibitor echothiophate iodide (Phospholine Iodide) are
more routinely used for this purpose. As might be expected, phy-

FIGURE 3.3
Structures of physostigmine (a naturally occurring AChE inhibitor) and three synthetic AChE inhibitors.

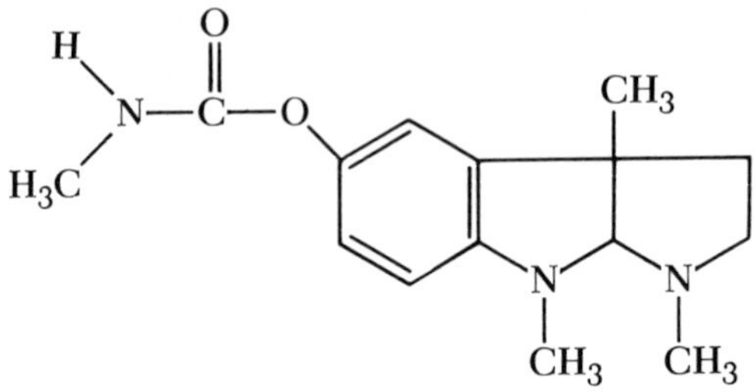

Physostigmine

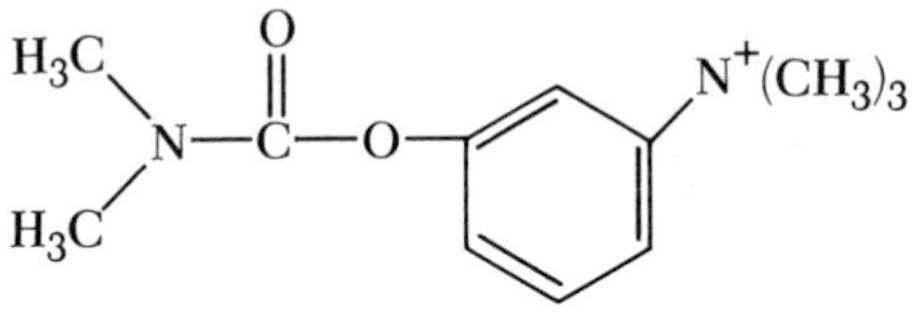

Neostigmine

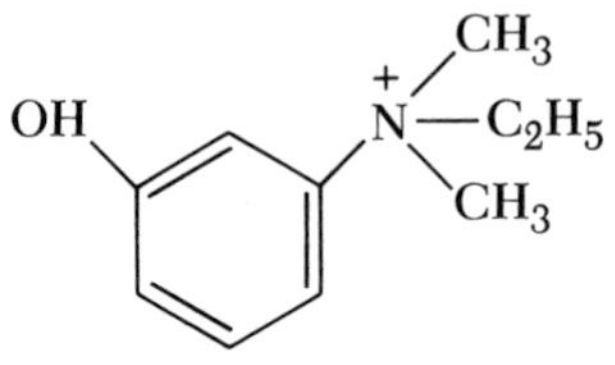

Edrophonium

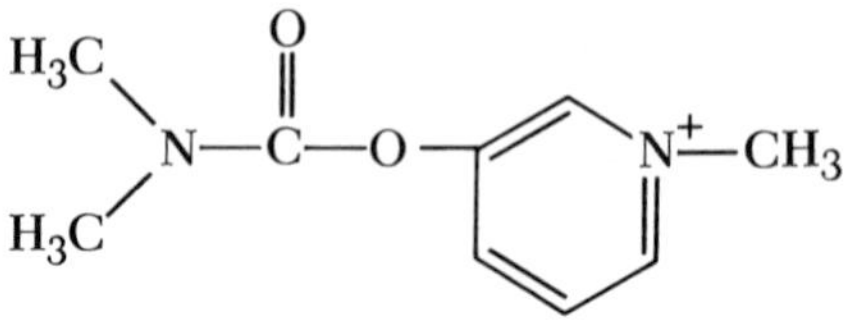

Pyridostigmine

sostigmine affects the gastrointestinal tract, stimulates gastric contractions, and increases the secretion of hydrochloric acid. At the neuromuscular junction, certain of these drugs are widely used to increase ACh levels at the termination of surgery to overcome the blockade of neuromuscular transmission produced by the neuromuscular blocking agents administered by the anesthesiologist. Physostigmine also is useful in the treatment of atropine poisoning (see p. 30).

Neostigmine (Prostigmin), pyridostigmine (Mestinon), and edrophonium (Tensilon) are additional reversible AChE inhibitors (Figure 3.3). Low doses of edrophonium also are used in the diagnosis of myasthenia gravis because in this disease it causes a brief augmentation of skeletal muscle contraction. Neostigmine and pyridostigmine are used for the long-term pharmacological management of this disease because their actions are more prolonged. Both serve as adjunctive therapy to steroid administration, removal of the thymus gland, and plasmapheresis—all of which are aimed at a presumed autoimmune etiology of myasthenia gravis.

IRREVERSIBLE AChE INHIBITORS

Before World War II, only the "reversible" AChE inhibitors were available; during the war, however, highly toxic compounds, the class *organophosphates*, were developed as chemical warfare agents. The toxicity of these compounds was due to their "irreversible" inactivation of AChE. Today, these agents have little therapeutic application and they are of interest principally because they are used widely as insecticides. As discussed above, the use of echothiophate iodide for the treatment of glaucoma is one exception.

The prototypical irreversible AChE inhibitor is a compound called diisopropylfluorophosphate (DFP) (Figure 3.4). DFP combines with the enzyme AChE, forms a stable phosphorylated enzyme, and permanently inhibits AChE activity unless a "reactivator" of the original AChE is given rapidly as an antidote (see below). Numerous other agents have been developed in addition

FIGURE 3.4
Structures of three "irreversible" AChE-inhibitors.

Diisopropyl fluorophosphate (DFP)

Parathion

Malathion

Echothiophate

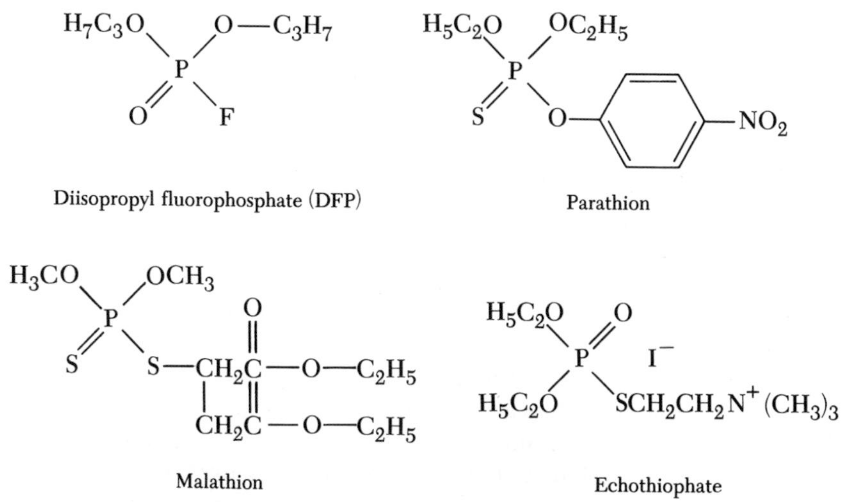

TABLE 3.1
Manifestations of poisoning with irreversible AChE inhibitors

Muscarinic symptoms	Nicotinic symptoms	CNS symptoms
Decreased heart rate	Muscle twitching	Tremors
Decreased blood pressure	Increased heart rate	Confusion
Pinpoint pupils	Muscle weakness	Staggering
Blurred vision		Restlessness
Increased tearing		Seizures
Salivation		Reduced respiration
Sweating		Cardiovascular failure
Bronchial constriction		Respiratory paralysis
Respiratory distress		

to DFP, such as the widely used insecticides malathion and parathion (Figure 3.4). "Nerve gases" include Sarin, Soman, and Tabun. Although the toxic manifestations of all these agents are listed in Table 3.1, respiratory failure is the usual cause of fatalities.

In the early 1950s, the compound pralidoxime was developed to dephosphorylate the enzyme and thus reactivate it. Pralidoxime is available in hospital emergency rooms in areas where insecticide poisoning occurs.

CHOLINERGIC BLOCKING AGENTS

Cholinergic blocking agents, also called *anticholinergic drugs*, are subdivided into those that block the actions of ACh at either nicotinic or muscarinic sites (Figure 3.5). The neuromuscular blocking agents such as curare and pancuronium (discussed next) are examples of nicotinic blockers; that is, they exert their actions at the nicotinic receptors at the neuromuscular junction. The nicotinic receptors at autonomic ganglia are blocked by drugs such as hexamethonium and trimethaphan (Arfonad), which produce an in-

FIGURE 3.5
Classification of cholinergic blocking agents.

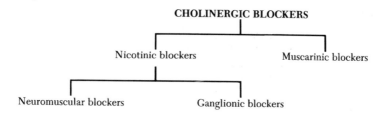

tense degree of hypotension as a result of relaxation of the smooth muscle of blood vessels. These agents are seldom used today since this effect can be achieved better by newer agents.

Anticholinergic drugs that preferentially block muscarinic receptors are termed *antimuscarinic drugs*. The belladonna alkaloids, atropine and scopolamine (Figure 3.6), are the prototypical agents of this group; both drugs have important uses in opthalmology, anesthesia, and certain cardiac and gastrointestinal disorders. They also serve as antidotes for the AChE inhibitors, protecting the muscarinic receptors from overstimulation by the excessive levels of ACh that may arise after inhibition of this enzyme.

Blockade of muscarinic receptors produces pupillary dilatation;

FIGURE 3.6
Structures of two alkaloids with cholinergic blocking activity at muscarinic receptor sites (antimuscarinic drugs).

$$H_2C—CH—CH_2$$
$$|\quad\quad|$$
$$NCH_3\ CH—O—CO—CH$$
$$|\quad\quad|$$
$$H_2C—CH—CH_2$$

$$CH_2OH$$
$$|$$
$$CH$$
$$|$$
$$C_6H_5$$

Atropine

$$HC—CH—CH_2$$
$$|\quad\quad|$$
$$O\quad NCH_6\ CH—O—CO—CH$$
$$|\quad\quad|$$
$$HC—CH—CH_2$$

$$CH_2OH$$
$$|$$
$$CH$$
$$|$$
$$C_6H_5$$

Scopolamine

TABLE 3.2
Effects of atropine in relation to dosage

Dose (mg)	Effects
0.5	Slight cardiac slowing; some dryness of mouth; inhibition of sweating
1	Definite dryness of mouth; thirst; acceleration of heart, sometimes preceded by slowing; mild dilatation of pupil
2.0	Rapid heart rate; palpitation; marked dryness of mouth; dilated pupils; some blurring of near vision
5	All the above symptoms marked; speech disturbed; difficulty in swallowing; restlessness and fatigue; headache; dry, hot skin; difficulty in micturition; reduced intestinal peristalsis
≥ 10	Above symptoms more marked; pulse rapid and weak; iris practically obliterated; vision very blurred; skin flushed, hot, dry, and scarlet; ataxia, restlessness, and excitement; hallucinations and delirium; coma

SOURCE: N. Weiner, "Atropine, Scopolamine, and Related Antimuscarinic Drugs," in A. G. Gilman, L. S. Goodman, T. W. Rall, and F. Murad (eds.), *The Pharmacological Basis of Therapeutics*, 7th ed., Macmillan, New York, 1985, p. 138.

increased conduction velocity of cardiac impulses, tachycardia; reduced bronchial, salivary, and sweat gland secretions (leading to dry mouth and dry skin); and reduced tone of visceral smooth muscle, which may result in gastric atony and urinary retention. They also may inhibit penile erection. Scopolamine also affects the CNS, producing sedation and amnesia. Overdoses of atropine or scopolamine can produce toxicities characterized by excitement and mania, hot and dry skin, dilated pupils, and tachycardia (Table 3.2). Physostigmine, as might be expected, is an antidote for atropine poisoning, just as atropine is an antidote for physostigmine overdose.

A large group of synthetic atropine derivatives are available and marketed for clinical use in the symptomatic relief of peptic ulcer disease.

Atropine and scopolamine also are used to relieve some symptoms of Parkinson's disease, a CNS disorder characterized by loss of dopamine neurons. In fact, such antimuscarinic agents frequently are combined with levodopa as part of the pharmacologic treatment of Parkinsonism.

NEUROMUSCULAR BLOCKING AGENTS

As shown in Figure 1.1, the efferent nerves are subdivided into motor, which innervate skeletal muscles, and autonomic. The cell bodies of these "motor neurons" originate in the ventral horn of the spinal cord; upon leaving the spinal cord, their axons innervate all the skeletal muscles. ACh is released from the nerve terminal after transmission of an electrical impulse down the axon of the motor neuron; this transmitter activates the postsynaptic receptors on the muscle fibers and initiates the process of muscle contraction.

The neuromuscular blocking agents exert their effects by blocking the postsynaptic receptors such that ACh released from the nerve terminals of motor neurons cannot initiate muscle contraction. Two types of neuromuscular blocking agents are available— depolarizing and nondepolarizing. Succinylcholine (Anectine) is the only depolarizing agent available, while there are six nondepolarizing agents (Table 3.3) currently marketed.

Succinylcholine (SCh) closely resembles ACh. As Figure 3.7 demonstrates, the SCh molecule is composed of two molecules of

TABLE 3.3
Characteristics of neuromuscular blocking drugs

Drug	Elimination half-life (min)	Metab- olized in liver (%)	Excreted unchanged in bile (%)	Excreted unchanged in urine (%)	Other (%)	Total (%)
D-Tubocurarine (Curare)	120	0	>50	<50	0	100
Pancuronium (Pavulon)	120	35	5	60	0	100
Gallamine (Flaxedil)	120	0	0	100	0	100
Metocurine (Metubine)	120	0	0	100	0	100
Atracurium (Tracrium)	30	0	0	0	100	100
Vercuronium (Norcuron)	75	0	40–50	5–10	50–60	100
Succinylcholine (Anectine)	2–3	0	0	0	100	100

All values are approximate and are intended to give the student a guide to understanding drug disposition and to appropriate selection of an agent for a particular patient.
SOURCE: Adapted from R. M. Julien, *Understanding Anesthesia*, Addison-Wesley, Palo Alto, CA, 1984.

FIGURE 3.7
Chemical structures of acetylcholine (ACh) and succinylcholine (SCh).

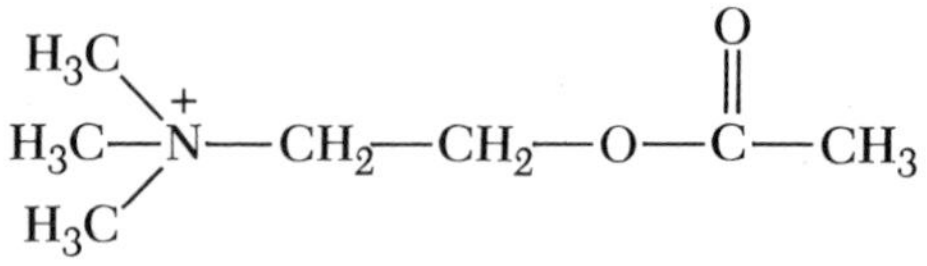

ACh

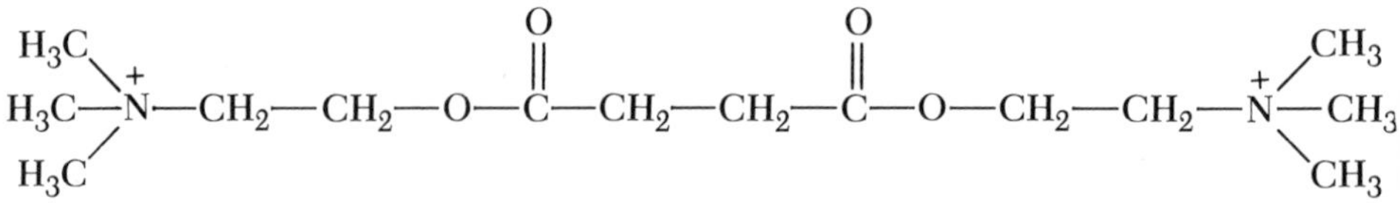

SCh

ACh bonded together. Though it activates (depolarizes) postsynaptic receptors in the same manner as does ACh, it also produces neuromuscular blockade at the same time. This is because SCh persists at the receptor for 3 to 5 minutes, much longer than the fraction of a second that ACh persists. SCh is a more complex structure than ACh and requires more time to be metabolized by plasma cholinesterase, an enzyme found in plasma. During this time, the postsynaptic receptors remain insensitive to ACh released from the nerve terminal. SCh is used primarily to produce a few minutes of profound muscle paralysis necessary for brief medical procedures that require such relaxation. The drug should be used only by medical experts and anesthesiologists trained in the management of patients in such a state of paralysis.

The *nondepolarizing* or *competitive* neuromuscular blocking agents exert a curarelike action and produce profound paralysis of neuromuscular transmission. They are administered in order to obtain the muscle relaxation necessary to conduct many surgical procedures. Each dose of tubocurarine, the prototype agent, produces muscle paralysis that persists for about 2 hours. Other nondepolarizing neuromuscular blockers with similar durations of action include pancuronium (Pavulon), metocurine (Metubine), and gallamine (Flaxedil). They differ primarily in their routes of metabolism and excretion. More recently, atracurium (Tracrium) and vercuronium (Norcuron), two agents with shorter durations of action (about 15 to 40 minutes) have become available.

All six of these drugs physically compete with ACh for the postsynaptic receptors on muscle cells and, if present in sufficient quantity, block access of ACh to the receptor—thus blocking transmission and producing paralysis. Termination of the neuromuscular blocking action of these six drugs depends on either (1) a reduced concentration of the drug at the neuromuscular junction, due to its metabolism or excretion (Table 3.3) or (2) increased concentrations of ACh such that increased amounts of it are available to compete for the receptors. This can be achieved by the administration of an AChE inhibitor. Such a drug will block the enzyme that metabolizes ACh and lead to increased availability of the transmitter to overcome the competitive blockade. AChE inhibitors used for this purpose include neostigmine, edrophonium, and pyridostigmine. To protect against the bradycardia produced by increasing ACh availability, an anticholinergic drug such as atropine or glycopyrrolate is co-administered.

Numerous factors will alter an individual's response to such drugs and the need for dosage alterations make medical expertise essential for their use.

READINGS

Julien, R. M., *Understanding Anesthesia*, Addison-Wesley, Palo Alto, CA, 1984.

Taylor, P., "Cholinergic Agonists" and "Anticholinesterase Agents," in A. G. Gilman, L. S. Goodman, T. W. Rall, and F. Murad (eds.), *The Pharmacological Basis of Therapeutics*, 7th ed., Macmillan, New York, 1985, pp. 100–129.

Vinderhoet, A. J., "The Role of the Parasympathetic Division of the Autonomic Nervous System in Stress and the Emotions," *Int. J. Psychosom.*, **32**:28–34 (1985).

CHAPTER 4

HISTAMINE, SEROTONIN, AND PROSTAGLANDINS

HISTAMINE AND ANTIHISTAMINIC DRUGS

Histamine (Figure 4.1), one of the most potent and widely distributed of the body's natural chemicals, is involved in a wide variety of physiologic processes, the most prominent of which is the response to allergic reactions and tissue injury. It has a function in gastric secretions and a possible role as a chemical transmitter within the CNS.

FIGURE 4.1
Chemical structure of histamine.

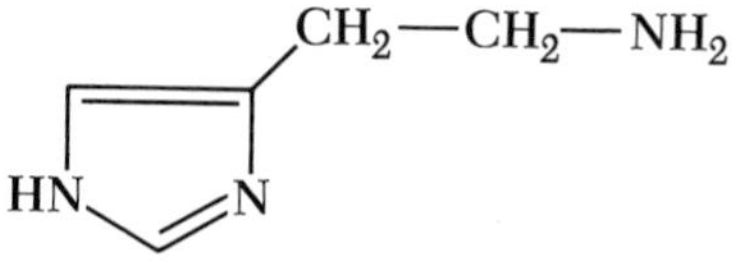

$$CH_2-CH_2-NH_2$$

Histamine acts on two types of specific receptors, H_1 and H_2. One of histamine's most prominent effects is contraction of the smooth muscle of the bronchi, which results in bronchoconstriction. This effect is mediated by H_1 receptors, which are readily blocked by the classical antihistamines such as diphenhydramine (Benadryl). Contraction of the gastrointestinal tract is also mediated by these H_1 receptors; as might be expected, such contraction is blocked by diphenhydramine.

Some effects of histamine cannot be blocked by the classical antihistamines but are susceptible to blockade by the newly developed H_2 blockers. H_2 receptors underlie the action of histamine in mediating secretion of stomach acid, and this action is blocked by the H_2 blockers cimetidine (Tagamet) and ranitidine (Zantac). Both H_1 and H_2 receptors apparently underlie the vasodilator effects of histamine, an effect that produces the severe drop in blood pressure following the massive release of histamine in the body (such as that which occurs in anaphylactic shock).

Histamine is found in highest concentrations in the lungs, skin, stomach, and the upper portion of the small intestine. Much of the body's histamine is located inside specialized cells such as the basophils (in blood) and the mast cells (in lungs, blood, stomach, and numerous other body tissues). In response to injury, to antigen-antibody reactions, and to a variety of drugs, histamine is released from its storage sites in basophils and mast cells and exerts its characteristic effects. Morphine and curare are two examples of drugs known to cause the release of histamine from mast cells, and each produces hypotension as a result.

The effect of histamine release on the cardiovascular system is vasodilatation and a fall in blood pressure proportional to the amount of histamine released. When evoked by an allergic, antigen-antibody, response, such release can produce very severe hypotension, which is often referred to as an anaphylactic response. As the capillaries of the skin dilate, a blush response is observed and the skin becomes hot and flushed. As a result of the increased permeability of the dilated venules, plasma proteins and water diffuse from the plasma to the extracellular space, which results in the formation of edema. The heart usually is not affected by histamine, and the fall in blood pressure is due almost entirely to vasodilatation.

Bronchial smooth muscle is intensely stimulated by histamine, which results in severe bronchoconstriction. In patients with asthma, such a reaction can be fatal. The asthmatic's response is so intense that antihistamines have little or no effect in ameliorating it, despite the fact that histamine-induced bronchoconstriction is mediated by H_1 receptors.

Histamine is a powerful stimulant of gastric hydrochloric acid secretion. This is because of histamine's direct effect on the glandular cells of the stomach and is not mediated entirely by the autonomic nervous system, even though surgical transection of the vagus nerve will further decrease acid release. Indeed, such surgery frequently is performed in patients with intractable peptic ulcer who do not respond adequately to H_2 blocking agents (see p. 39) as well as in patients undergoing partial removal of the stomach.

Histamine is released in response to skin irritation such as cuts and insect bites, and it causes local reddening, a red "flare," and a wheal of edema (the so-called triple response of Lewis). These effects are the result of local vasodilatation and increased capillary permeability.

INHIBITOR OF HISTAMINE RELEASE

In patients exquisitly sensitive to the physiologic effects of histamine, antihistaminic drugs (i.e., drugs which compete with histamine for its receptors) may be only partially effective. Cromolyn, however, is an agent that inhibits the release of histamine from mast cells in response to antigen-antibody reactions. This agent is useful in the prophylactic management of certain cases of asthma and severe allergic states. Cromolyn acts directly on the mast cells of the lungs, decreasing the stimulus for producing bronchospasm. It is not effective when taken orally, so it is usually inhaled as a powder through the nostrils. A portion of this inhaled powder is taken into the lungs and is therapeutically effective. That which is absorbed into the bloodstream from the lungs is excreted unchanged in both urine and bile. It should be noted that Cromolyn is used only in the prophylactic treatment of asthma; it is not effective in the treatment of an acute asthmatic attack.

H_1 RECEPTOR ("CLASSICAL") ANTIHISTAMINES

The actions of histamine on bronchial and vascular smooth muscle can be blocked by the H_1 receptor antihistamines. Diphenhydramine (Benadryl) and tripelennamine (Pyribenzamine) were two of the first H_1 blockers introduced into medicine. These and other H_1 blockers (Figure 4.2) exert a competitive, reversible blockade of H_1 receptors. The names, doses, and side effects of several H_1 blockers are listed in Table 4.1. Most of these drugs are taken orally. Drowsiness, the most common side effect, often limits daily use and dosage. However, such sedation may be used to therapeutic advantage, since antihistamines with a high degree of sedation often make excellent bedtime sedatives, especially when insomnia is complicated by nasal congestion. Other, less frequent, side effects usually involve some degree of atropinelike action that results in dry mouth and some minor blurring of vision. Primary uses of H_1 receptor antihistamines involve the symptomatic treatment of such allergies as urticaria, seasonal rhinitis, and conjunctivitis and the prevention

TABLE 4.1
Drugs, doses, and side effects of selected H_1 antihistimines

Name	Trade name	Range of daily dose (mg/day)	Sedative properties	Anticholinergic properties
Brompheniramine	Dimetane	8–24	+ +	+
Carbinoxamine	Clistin	12–24	+ +	+ +
Chlorpheniramine	Chlor-Trimeton	8–24	+ +	+
Cyclizine*	Marezine	100–200	+	+ +
Cyproheptadine	Periactin	8–20	+ +	+
Dimenhydrinate*	Dramamine	100–200	+ + +	+ +
Diphenhydramine	Benadryl	50–150	+ + +	+ +
Meclizine*	Antivert, Bonine	25–150	+	+ +
Promethazine	Phenergan	25–37.5	+ + +	+ +
Pyrilamine	Neo-Antergan	75–150	+ +	+
Terfenadine	Seldane	60–120	0†	+
Tripelennamine	Pyribenzamine, PBZ	50–200	+ + +	+ +
Triprolidine	Actidil	5–10	+ +	+

* Primarily used for prevention of motion sickness.
† Does not cross the blood-brain barrier to cause CNS sedation.

FIGURE 4.2
Basic structure of "classical" antihistamines ("x," "R$_1$," and "R$_2$" are sites of substitution) and several widely used antihistamines. Terfenadine does not share this basic structure.

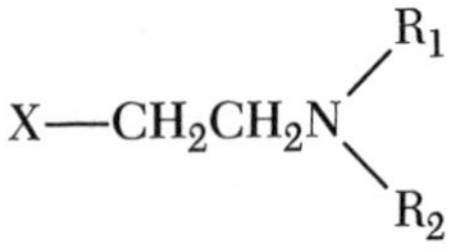

Basic structure

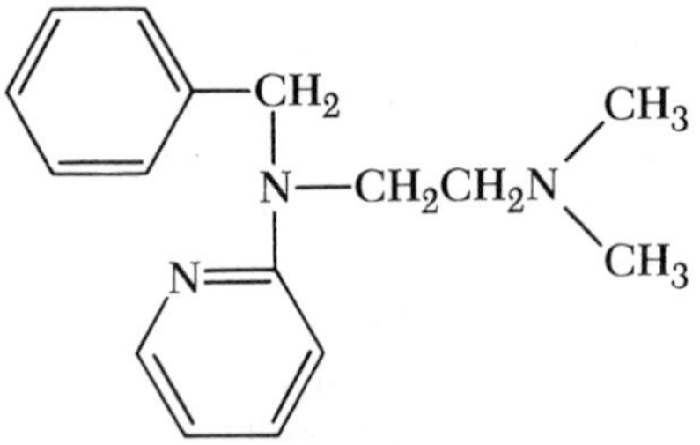

Tripelennamine
(Pyribenzamine)

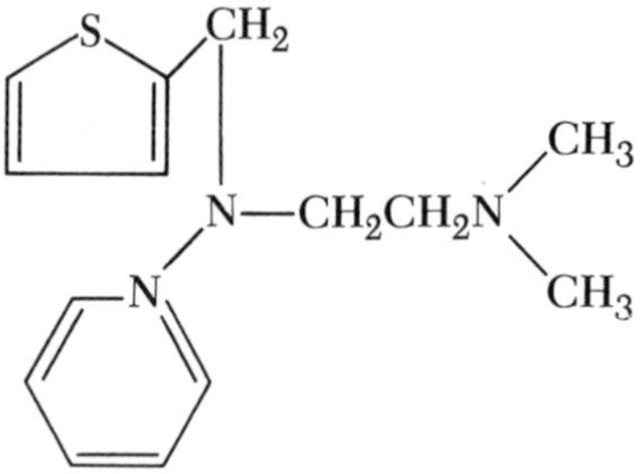

Methapyrilene
(Histadil)

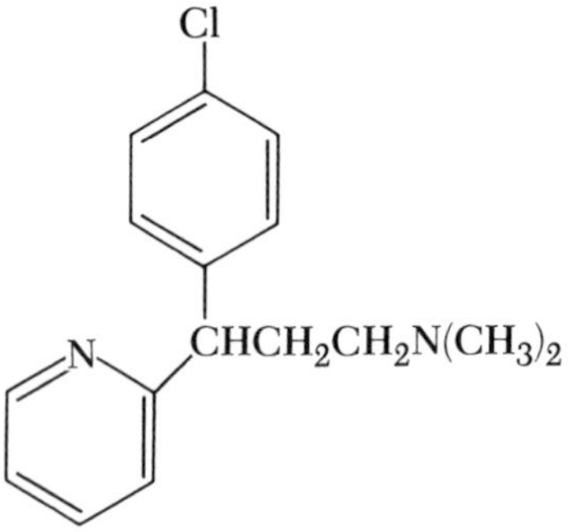

Chlorpheniramine
(Chlor-Trimeton)

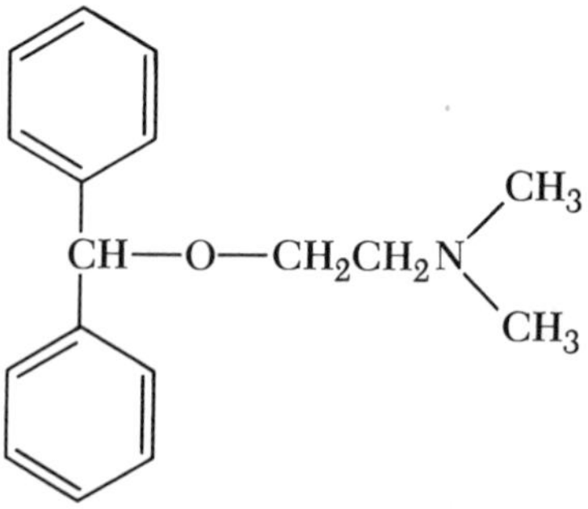

Diphenhydramine
(Benadryl)

FIGURE 4.2. (*continued*)

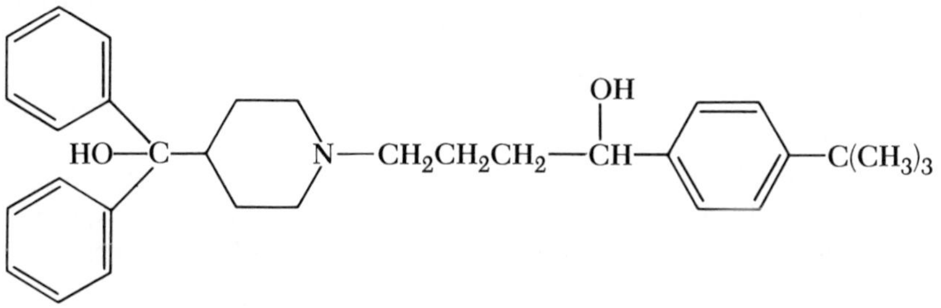

Terfenadine
(Seldane)

of motion sickness. Antihistamines have no antiviral effects and are of little or no use in treating the common cold.

H₂ RECEPTOR ANTIHISTAMINES

Because the H_1 receptor blockers do not block the effects of histamine on gastric acid secretion, an extensive search was made for safe and effective blockers of H_2 receptors. This search led to the introduction of cimetidine (Tagamet) and, more recently, ranitidine (Zantac). Both drugs (Figure 4.3) are quite selective for H_2 receptors

FIGURE 4.3
Structures of H₂ blockers.

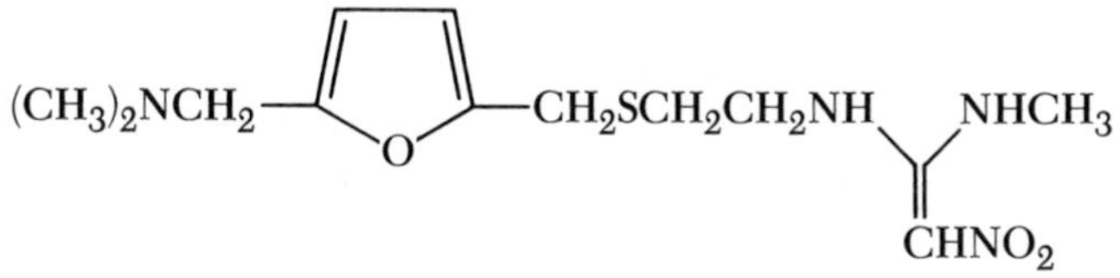

Ranitidine
(Zantac)

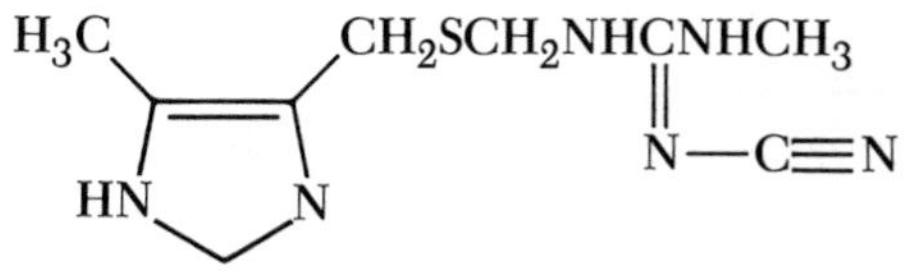

Cimetidine
(Tagamet)

and have little or no affinity for H_1 receptors. They reduce both the volume of gastric secretions and the amount of hydrochloric acid contained within these secretions. Their degree of efficacy is related to the dose administered. Both drugs are quite well absorbed when taken orally, and are now also available in parenteral form as well.

Side effects of these drugs are rare. Sedation is not a problem, because these drugs do not penetrate into the CNS. Rarely has cimetidine been associated with depression of drug-metabolizing enzymes in the liver, and this factor may be important in certain drug interactions. Ranitidine has a longer duration of action than cimetidine and is often given only twice daily, as opposed to at least three times daily for cimetidine. Long-term experience with ranitidine on hepatic metabolism of other drugs is not yet complete.

SEROTONIN AND THE SEROTONIN ANTAGONISTS

The role of serotonin (Figure 4.4) in the body is unclear. It is almost certainly a transmitter within the brain, and it is found in the intestine and in smooth muscle. It is also widely distributed throughout the animal and plant kingdom. A variety of psychedelic drugs, such as LSD, are chemically related to serotonin; their psychedelic actions are thought to be secondary to drug-induced alterations in central serotonin synapses.

In the peripheral nervous system, serotonin resembles histamine—both cause vasodilatation, especially affecting the cerebral blood vessels, stimulate the intestine, and cause bronchoconstriction.

Serotonin antagonists include LSD, a psychedelic; methysergide, a compound useful in the prevention of migraine headache; and several ergot alkaloids. Examples of the latter include ergotamine (Gynergen), ergonovine (Ergotrate), and methylergonovine (Methergine). Methysergide (Sansert), which blocks the vasodilator properties of serotonin, is useful for the prophylactic treatment of migraine headaches. The drug effect may take 1 to 2 days to develop, and the drug is without effect in terminating acute attacks of migraine. The ergot alkaloids are potent stimulants of smooth muscle, particularly that of blood vessels and the uterus.

Ergonovine and methylergonovine are used in obstetrics to induce postpartum uterine contractions. Ergotamine is widely used in the treatment of migraine headaches because of its vasoconstrictive actions on intracranial blood vessels. Serious side effects as-

FIGURE 4.4

Structures of serotonin and three antiserotonin drugs that have widely differing actions, despite structural similarity.

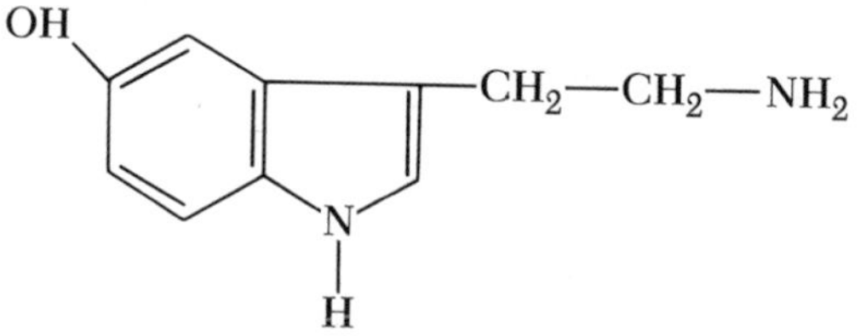

Serotonin

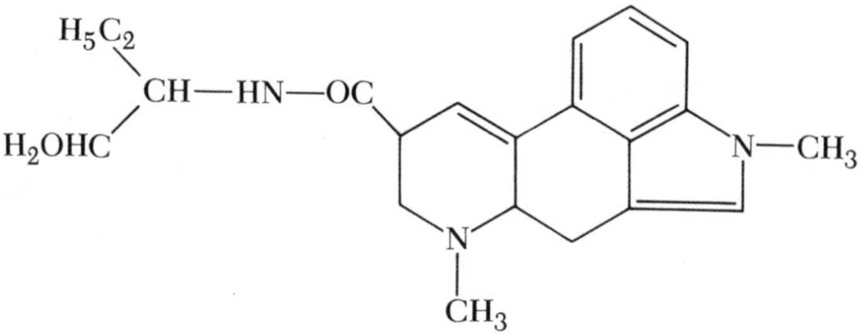

Methysergide
(Sansert)

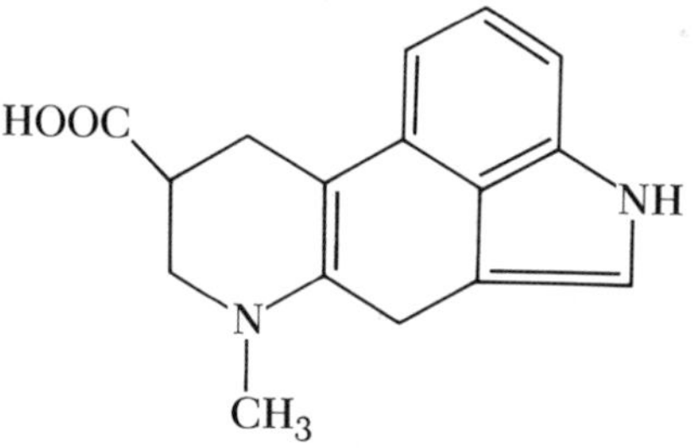

Lysergic acid

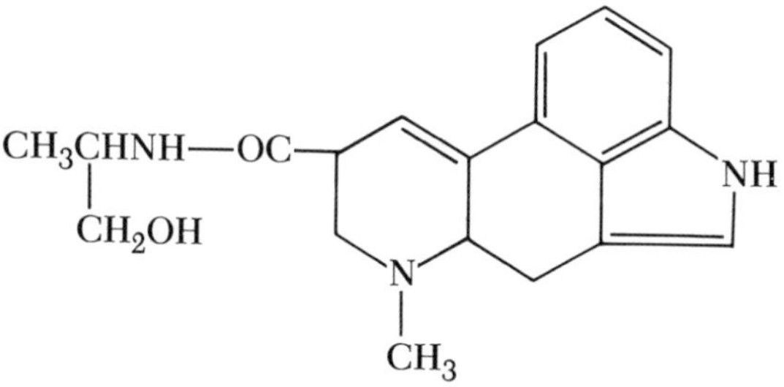

Ergonovine
(Ergotrate)

sociated with the use of methylsergide and the ergot alkaloids primarily involve vasoconstriction of the peripheral arterioles supplying the extremities. Such reduced blood flow may lead to gangrene, especially in patients with peripheral vascular disease. Hypertension is also aggravated. In addition, fibrosis affecting the lungs and the urinary tract has been reported with methysergide. Obviously, close physician guidance is essential with these agents.

PROSTAGLANDINS

The prostaglandins have received wide attention during the last 2 decades. These acidic lipids (fats) (Figure 4.5) are found in virtually every tissue and body fluid. They exert profound effects on many organ functions, and blockade of their effects underlies the mechanism of action of anti-inflammatory analgesics such as aspirin. Prostaglandins are used to induce labor, as abortifacients, and for a variety of other clinical uses. Numerous prostaglandins have been synthesized or identified, including PGE_1, PGE_2, PGF_1, PGF_2, and others. The prostaglandins exert various effects, and one may

FIGURE 4.5
Structure of two representative prostaglandins.

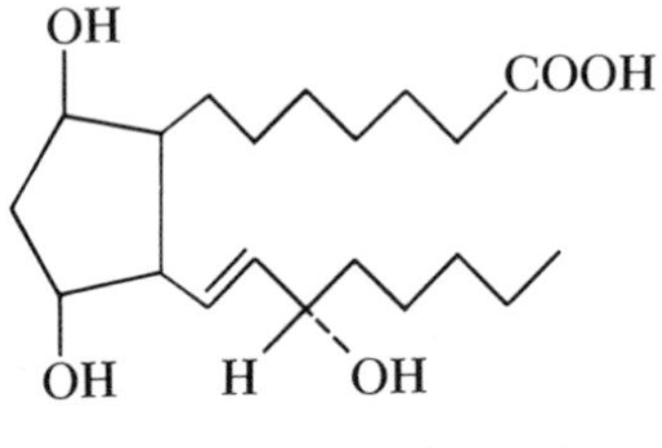

Prostaglandin $F_{1\alpha}$ ($PGF_{1\alpha}$)

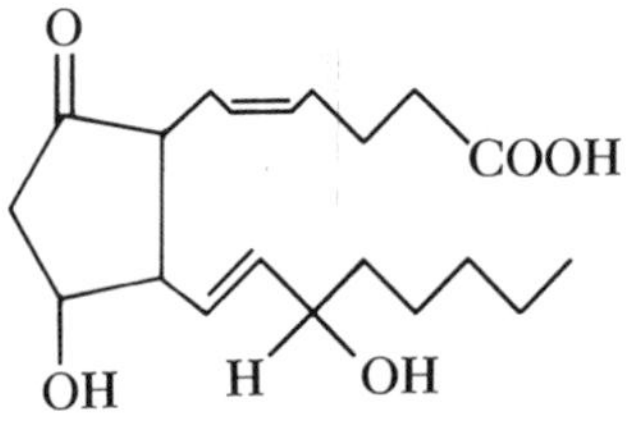

Prostaglandin E_2 (PGE_2)

actually counteract the effects of another. For example, PGE is a bronchodilator and PGF is a bronchoconstrictor. Several prostaglandins are uterine stimulants.

Prostaglandins also may be involved in inflammatory responses. Indomethacin (Indocin), ibuprofen (Motrin), and aspirin all block the synthesis of prostaglandins and, indeed, the anti-inflammatory actions of these drugs may follow from drug-induced inhibition of prostaglandin synthesis. Much remains to be learned about the physiologic role of prostaglandins and any disease associated with their excesses or deficiencies in the body. Prostaglandin research is new, exciting, and filled with promise.

READINGS

American Medical Association, "Histamine and Antihistamines," in *AMA Drug Evaluations*, 6th ed., American Medical Association, Chicago, 1986, pp. 1041–1048.

Beaven, M. S., *Histamine: Its Role in Physiological and Pathological Processes*, S. Karger, Basel, 1978.

Douglas, W. W., "Histamine and 5-hydroxytryptamine (Serotonin) and their Antagonists," in A. G. Gilman, L. S. Goodman, T. W. Rall, and F. Murad (eds.), *The Pharmacological Basis of Therapeutics*, 7th ed., Macmillan, New York, 1985, pp. 605–638.

Estelle, F., R. Simons, and K. J. Simmons, "Pharmacologic Treatment of Rhinitis," *Clin. Rev. Allergy*, 2:237–253 (1984).

Marquardt, D. L., "Histamine," *Clin. Rev. Allergy*, 1:343–351 (1983).

Paskin, N. H., "Pharmacology of Migraine," *Ann. Rev. Pharmacol. Toxicol.*, 21:463–478 (1981).

Salvaggio, J. E. (ed.), "Primer on Allergic and Immunologic Diseases," *J. Amer. Med. Assoc.*, 248:2579–2772 (1982).

Sorkin, E. M., and R. C. Heel, "Terfenadine. A Review of its Pharmacodynamic Properties and Therapeutic Efficacy," *Drugs*, 1:34–56 (1985).

DRUGS USED FOR CARDIAC
AND VASCULAR DISORDERS

CHAPTER 5

THE HEART IN HEALTH AND DISEASE

This chapter initiates a six-chapter discussion on the heart, disorders of cardiac function, and the treatment of these disorders by pharmacologic agents. Cardiac disorders can be divided into the following four general areas (Table 5.1):

1. Failure of the heart to pump adequate quantities of blood
2. Altered conduction of electrical impulses resulting in cardiac arrythmias
3. Reduced or restricted flow of blood through the coronary arteries
4. Altered function of one or more of the four heart valves

TABLE 5.1
Overview of disorders of cardiac function and relevant terms applied

Cardiac disorders	Terms applied
1. Failure to pump adequate quantities of blood to meet the needs of body tissues	Heart failure Congestive heart failure
2. Disorders of the electrical conductive system	Cardiac arrhythmias (various) Heart block Ectopic foci Flutter/fibrillation
3. Reduction or obstruction to the flow of blood in the coronary arteries	Atherosclerotic coronary artery disease Angina pectoris Myocardial infarction, if reduced flow leads to muscle death
4. Altered function of one or more of the four heart valves	Valvular stenosis Valvular insufficiency (incompetence, regurgitation)

While valvular disorders are usually correctable by surgery, the other cardiac disorders are amenable to pharmacologic treatment. Before initiating discussion of the pharmacologic treatment of cardiac disorders, however, we must first understand certain aspects of cardiac function, both in the healthy heart and in the failing heart.

THE HEART AS A PUMP

The only purpose of the heart is to provide the body with sufficient flow of blood to carry oxygen and nutrients to body tissues and to remove waste products. Thus, blood flow is directly dependent on the ability of the heart to pump blood and, together with autonomic regulation of blood vessel tone, to maintain an adequate blood pressure within the systemic circulation. When the heart fails to function adequately as a pump, its ability to propel blood forward into the arteries is impeded, blood pressure falls, blood flow to body tissues declines, and blood collects in pools in the large central veins and in the lungs.

The heart is indeed a marvelous pump. Usually weighing less than 1 pound and pumping at a rate of about 70 beats per minute, the heart beats over 100,000 times a day, 36 million times a year, or about 2.5 billion times in a normal life span. At a normal output of about 70 milliliters (ml) [slightly over 2 ounces (oz)] per beat, the heart pumps over 1800 gallons (gal) of blood a day. The amount of blood pumped in a lifetime is staggering.

Cardiac output refers to the amount of blood pumped by the heart per minute. Cardiac output is determined by the following equation

$$Cardiac\ output\ =\ stroke\ volume\ \times\ heart\ rate$$

Stroke volume is the amount of blood pumped by the heart per beat (about 70 ml in a normal adult) and the heart rate is the number of heart beats per minute (usually about 70). Thus, cardiac output in a normal adult is about 4900 ml, or 4.9 liters (1), per minute.

FUNCTIONAL ANATOMY

The heart is a four-chambered pump composed of two atria, two ventricles, and four one-way valves (Figure 5.1). Venous blood returns to the heart in the vena cava, the largest vein in the body. The superior vena cava returns blood to the heart from the head and upper extremities, and the inferior vena cava returns blood from the trunk and lower extremities. The venous blood enters the heart through the right atrium. The right atrium functions primarily as an entryway for venous blood into the right ventricle, but it also pumps weakly to help fill the right ventricle. On the surface of the right atrium is a structure called the sinoatrial node (SA node); it is here that the cardiac electrical impulse originates (see pp. 52–54). Blood enters the right ventricle from the right atrium by passing through the tricuspid valve. Like the other three heart valves, this valve functions as a one-way valve to prevent blood from flowing backwards, in this case from the right ventricle back into the right atrium as the right ventricle contracts. The right ventricle is larger and more muscular than the right atrium but less so than the left ventricle. Mechanical contraction of the right ventricle forces blood forward through the pulmonic valve into the pulmonary artery, through the lung capillaries into the pulmonary veins, and, finally, through the veins into the left atrium. The right ventricle is less muscular than the left ventricle because the right ventricle pumps into a low-pressure circulation in the lungs [22/10 millimeters of mercury (mmHg)] while the left ventricle must pump against the high pressure systemic circulation (120/70 mmHg).

FIGURE 5.1
Structure of the heart, and course of blood flow through the heart chambers.
(From A. C. Guyton, *Textbook of Medical Physiology*, 7th ed., Saunders, Philadelphia, 1986.)

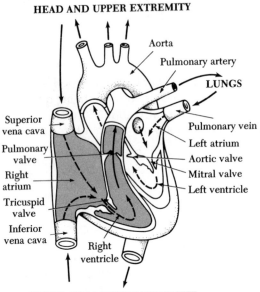

In the lungs, carbon dioxide diffuses from the blood into the air spaces of the alveoli and is replaced in the blood by oxygen. When carbon dioxide is exhaled, the oxygenated blood leaves the lungs in the pulmonary veins, enters the heart through the left atrium, and passes through the mitral valve into the left ventricle. When the left ventricle contracts, blood is pumped through the aortic valve into the aorta. Blood in the aorta flows forward through smaller and smaller arteries, finally reaching the capillary beds within body tissues; here oxygen is given up to the tissues and carbon dioxide diffuses back into blood. This deoxygenated blood then enters the venules and progresses into the veins and returns to the heart in the superior and inferior vena cava, and the cycle is repeated.

Since the left ventricle must pump against the highest pressures (a systolic pressure of about 120 mmHg in an adult with normal blood pressure), the greatest force of contraction in the heart is generated in the muscle surrounding the left ventricle. The major feature of heart failure is the inability of the left ventricle to generate enough force to pump against these high pressures in the systemic circulation. The existence of hypertension places additional burden

DRUGS USED FOR CARDIAC AND VASCULAR DISORDERS

on the left ventricle and increases the work it must perform. This increased work must be accompanied by increased blood flow to the muscle of the left ventricle (through the coronary arteries) in order to meet the increased metabolic needs of oxygen and nutrients. Failure of the muscle of the left ventricle to receive the required oxygen and nutrients can result in signs of cardiac *ischemia* as manifested by *angina pectoris* or ultimately by a heart attack (*myocardial infarction*). Failure of the left ventricle to pump adequate amounts of blood into the systemic circulation also results in increased pressure within the left ventricle and, ultimately, in the backwards transmission of this increased pressure into the pulmonary circulation. Once this happens, water is forced from the pulmonary vessels into the tissues of the lungs, resulting in pulmonary edema. Pulmonary edema occurs secondary to the failure of the left ventricle and is one symptom of *congestive heart failure* (CHF).

One of the major factors determining the amount of blood pumped by the heart each minute is the rate of blood flow into the heart from the vena cava. This is called *venous return*. The heart automatically pumps the total venous return forward through the pulmonary circulation and then into the systemic arteries so that blood can flow through the circuit again. Thus, the heart adapts itself almost instantaneously to widely varying inputs of blood into the right atrium. Such input depends on the requirements of the various tissues of the body and can vary between 4 or 5 l of blood pumped per minute to rates as high as 25 l or more per minute, such as might occur during strenuous exercise. Thus, within limits, the normal heart is capable of pumping all the blood that comes into it. Failure of the heart to perform this function is termed *heart failure*, and CHF commonly results.

The mechanism underlying this ability of the heart to vary its pumping ability in response to varied amounts of returned blood is as follows. When the cardiac muscle becomes stretched, as when extra amounts of blood enter the heart chambers, the muscle fibers become stretched and the muscle contracts with a greatly increased force, thereby automatically pumping this extra blood into the arteries. Thus, cardiac muscle, like skeletal muscle, has the ability to contract with increased force when the muscle is stretched. This is referred to as the *Frank-Starling law of the heart*.

ALTERED FUNCTION OF THE HEART VALVES

As stated above, the four heart valves function as one-way conduits directing the flow of blood through the four heart chambers and through the pulmonary and systemic systems. Flow of adequate amounts of blood in a forward direction depends upon two functions of the valve. The first is its ability to open wide enough to permit adequate amounts of blood to flow through these narrow orifices within the time period (less than 1 second) allowed for ventricular filling before each cardiac contraction. The second is its ability to close tightly during ventricular contraction so that there is a forward flow of blood with no backflow (regurgitation) into the atria from which the blood came. A heart valve that becomes scarred so that it fails to open properly is referred to as *stenotic*. Stenosis of the mitral valve may occur as a consequence of rheumatic fever. Failure of the valve to close completely during contraction, as in a failing or dilated heart, produces an incompetent valve, referred to as valvular insufficiency. Thus, in instances of aortic valve insufficiency, part of the blood that flowed from the left ventricle into the aorta during cardiac contraction flows backwards (regurgitates) from the aorta into the left ventricle during the time period of left ventricular filling. This reduces the efficiency of the heart as a forward pump.

Valvular stenosis and insufficiency are seldom treatable by pharmacologic agents. Surgical intervention may be necessary when a valvular disorder interferes with a person's ability to function normally in states of either resting or exercising. Valvular diseases may be detected with the aid of a stethoscope, since stenotic or incompetent valves produce turbulence in blood flow through the affected valve, resulting in an audible murmur.

ELECTRICAL EXCITATION OF THE HEART

In order to coordinate the proper sequence of contractions of the heart chambers, the heart contains special systems that generate rhythmic impulses capable of producing rhythmic contractions of the heart muscle. Many disorders of the heart are the result of alterations in the functioning of this excitatory and conduction system. Most of these disorders are amenable to pharmacologic treatment (see Chapter 7). The present discussion will outline the normal anatomic and physiologic mechanisms involved in this system and present a few of the most common disorders that result in cardiac arrhythmias. The cardiac electrical system is illustrated in Figure 5.2.

The *sinoatrial (SA) node* is formed by a group of specialized muscle cells and is located over the right atrium near the entrance

FIGURE 5.2
The SA node and the Purkinje system of the heart, showing also the AV node, the atrial internodal pathways, and the ventricular bundle branches. (From A. C. Guyton, *Textbook of Medical Physiology*, 7th ed., Saunders, Philadelphia, 1986.)

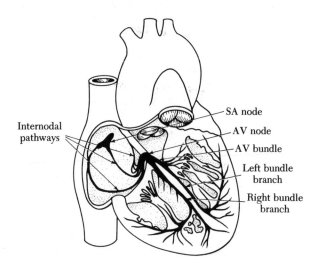

of the superior vena cava. It is the site of origin of the normal rhythmic impulses that are then propagated over the heart and result in cardiac contraction. Cells in the SA node depolarize spontaneously at a more rapid rate than those in other areas of the heart and because they thus control heart rate, they are called *pacemaker cells*. The electrical impulse for each cardiac contraction normally arises in the SA node, and the heart is said to be in *sinus rhythm*. The wave of depolarization that originates in the SA node spreads passively over the atrium, rapidly reaching another specialized group of cells that form the *atrioventricular (AV node)*. Cells of the AV node lie approximately at the junction of the right atrium and right ventricle. The AV node gives rise to a group of specialized muscle fibers (termed the *bundle of HIS*) which run from the AV node downward within the septum that separates the right and left ventricles. This bundle eventually branches into two separate bundles of conducting fibers, the *right* and *left bundles*. These eventually divide into finer and finer branches that ramify extensively throughout the ventricular muscle, exciting all muscle cells.

If the rate of depolarization of cells of the SA node slows, the pacemaker site of the heart shifts to the AV node, which contains the next most rapidly depolarizing cells of the heart. When this occurs, the heart is said to be in *nodal rhythm*.

The normal spread of electrical activity over and throughout the heart therefore occurs in the following sequence:

1. The cells of the SA node depolarize spontaneously
2. Electrical activity spreads over the surface of the right atrium, reaching the AV node
3. The electrical impulse is conducted through the AV node to the fibers of the bundle of HIS
4. Electrical impulses are conducted down the bundle to the right and left bundle branches, and then to the muscle cells of the ventricles
5. The ventricular muscles contract
6. After contraction the muscle cells "repolarize" so that they can be depolarized again when the next impulse arrives

The rate of depolarization of the SA node is both spontaneous and under the influence of both the sympathetic and parasympathetic divisions of the autonomic nervous system. Stimulation of the *vagus nerve*, which carries mostly parasympathetic fibers, releases acetylcholine onto the cells of the SA node and slows its rate of depolarization. This effect produces a bradycardia and slows impulse transmission through the node, thus reducing transmission of electrical impulses between the atria and the ventricles.

Sympathetic stimulation has the opposite effects on the heart, that is, impulse generation at the SA node and heart rate are both increased. Sympathetic stimulation also increases cardiac excitability and the force of contraction, which thus prepares the heart to increase its output of blood in response to exercise.

ABNORMAL CARDIAC RHYTHMS

The normal cardiac rhythm is said to be *sinus*, that is, originating in the SA node. Any other rhythm is said to be abnormal (Table 5.2). As stated above, if the rate of depolarization of AV nodal cells exceeds that of SA nodal cells, impulse generation commences in the AV node and the heart is said to be in *nodal rhythm*. Although this is usually of little functional significance, individuals who have failing hearts and depend upon atrial contractions to provide a "kick" to aid in ventricular filling may experience deleterious effects when the heart goes into nodal rhythm. Other arrhythmias are said to be (1) either atrial or ventricular in origin, (2) indicative of

TABLE 5.2
Cardiac dysrhythmias and their significance

Cardiac rhythms	Origin of impulse	Functional significance
Normal sinus rhythm	SA node	Normal
Sinus bradycardia	SA node	None if cardiac output is normal
Sinus tachycardia	SA node	Usually none unless concurrent coronary artery disease results in angina
Nodal rhythm	AV node	Loss of atrial "kick"
Premature atrial contractions	Atrial muscle	Usually innocuous
Premature ventricular contractions	Ventricular muscle	May be benign, or may increase risk of sudden death
Right bundle branch block	Conduction block in bundle fibers	May be innocuous
Left bundle branch block	Conduction block in bundle fibers	More serious; may require pacemaker
Atrial flutter	Atrial muscle	Requires intervention to reduce ventricular rate or to convert to sinus rhythm
Atrial fibrillation	Atrial muscle	Same as atrial flutter
Ventricular flutter	Ventricular muscle	Requires cardioversion
Ventricular fibrillation	Ventricular muscle	Fatal unless rapidly cardioverted

blockade at different points in the conduction of electrical impulses through the heart (i.e., blockade at the AV node or in the bundle of HIS), or (3) consisting of spontaneously generated abnormal impulses in either the atria or the ventricles. Common arrhythmias include (1) premature contractions caused by non-SA or non-AV nodal electrical foci in the atria or ventricles (*premature atrial contractions* or *premature ventricular contractions*), (2) *heart block* (blockade of transmission in the conductive system, most commonly occurring at the AV node or in one of the two branches of the bundle of HIS), and (3) *flutter* or *fibrillation* of either the atria or the ventricles. Flutter or fibrillation occur when either the atria or the ventricles begin to contract very rapidly, often incoordinately. The significance and treatment of cardiac arrhythmias are discussed in Chapter 7.

RESTRICTED CORONARY BLOOD FLOW

Blood is supplied to the heart muscle through the *coronary* circulation (Figure 5.3). Obstruction or restriction of flow through the coronary arteries results in approximately one-third of all deaths. To avoid ischemia of heart muscle, and ultimately to avoid infarction of an area of cardiac muscle, the coronary circulation must supply all the oxygen and nutrients required by the heart muscle at any given level of activity. Thus, when cardiac output requirement is increased or when the work load required by the heart muscle is increased, coronary blood flow must increase, that is, the coronary arteries must dilate, to provide the necessary oxygen requirements.

The coronary arteries, including the two main ones—the left and the right—originate at the base of the aorta just outside the aortic valve. The left coronary artery passes over the surface of the left ventricle, supplying most of the blood to this structure; the right coronary artery supplies blood to the right ventricle. Occlusion of the left coronary artery is especially disastrous since such occlusion severely impairs the pumping ability of this high-pressure, thick-walled chamber. Because the right ventricle pumps into a low-pressure system, it does not require the same amount of oxygen and is more tolerant of reductions in blood flow. Branches from the right coronary artery supply the cells of the SA and AV nodes. Damage to these branches can produce severe arrhythmias.

FIGURE 5.3
The coronary vessels. (From A. C. Guyton, *Textbook of Medical Physiology*, 7th ed., Saunders, Philadelphia, 1986.)

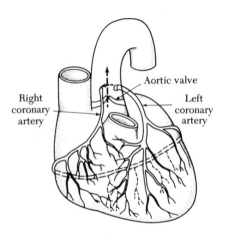

The coronary arteries and their small branches are innervated by the sympathetic nervous system, and increased sympathetic activity produces dilatation of coronary arteries with a resulting increase in coronary blood flow. This is consistent with the role of the SNS in preparing the body for exertion. In addition to sympathetic stimulation, coronary blood vessels can autoregulate and increase the flow of blood as myocardial oxygen demands are increased. Such autoregulation is accomplished through some as yet unidentified local influences.

Inadequate coronary blood flow frequently necessitates treatment. Surgical innervation by means of coronary artery bypass grafts is indicated when the bypassing of demonstrated points of localized mechanical obstruction will result in blood flow sufficient to meet oxygen requirements. Other techniques of relieving localized areas of coronary artery obstruction include dilatation (balloon angioplasty) and high-energy burning of the calcium deposits causing the obstruction (laser angioplasty). Pharmacologic intervention is used to reduce the need for increased coronary blood flow, by reducing blood pressure and heart rate, or to dilate coronary arteries. Drugs providing such benefits are discussed in Chapter 8.

READINGS

Braunwald, E. (ed.), *Heart Disease: A Textbook of Cardiovascular Medicine*, Saunders, Philadelphia, 1984.

Guyton, A. C., *Textbook of Medical Physiology*, Saunders, Philadelphia, 1986, pp. 150–204.

Hurst, J. W. (ed.), *The Heart*, McGraw-Hill, New York, 1982.

CHAPTER 6

DRUGS USED FOR HEART FAILURE

Heart failure refers to the heart's inability to pump sufficient quantities of blood to meet the demands of the body tissues. Characteristics of heart failure include a *decreased contractility* of the cardiac muscle, a reduced cardiac output, and higher-than-normal pressures in either the left or the right atrium as forward failure of pumping leads to increased backward pressure.

This serious illness affects 3 million Americans, and each year about 250,000 new cases are reported. Hypertension, the predominant precursor, and coronary artery disease are the two most frequent causes of heart failure. Because hypertension precedes cardiac failure in approximately 75 percent of patients, its early detection and control should greatly reduce the incidence of heart failure. The control of hypertension is discussed in Chapter 8.

Heart failure is accompanied by decreased strength of heart muscle contraction. As contractile strength is lost, cardiac output falls and several of the body's compensatory responses come into play. Reduced cardiac output leads to increased activity of the sympathetic nervous system—causing an increase in heart rate, force of contraction, and total peripheral resistance—and reduced blood flow to the kidneys. The increase in peripheral vascular resistance places additional load on the left ventricle, which can further aggravate the heart failure. Reduced perfusion of the kidneys leads to the secretion of aldosterone from the adrenal cortex (see Chapter 14), which causes water retention and plasma volume expansion.

The combination of reduced cardiac output, increased plasma volume, and reduced venous return leads to the formation of edema, especially in the lungs (congestive heart failure) and the lower extremities. Thus, breathing may become difficult and the ankles may become swollen.

One result of heart failure is that the ability of cardiac muscle to respond to the needs of exercise or exertion is greatly decreased. The Frank-Starling law of the heart states that, within limits, the force of cardiac contraction increases as heart muscle is stretched. The heart dilates and the muscle fibers stretch as a result of the increased blood volume in the ventricles at the end of contraction. According to the Frank-Starling law, as long as the heart can dilate further, it can increase its output (Figure 6.1a). Such compensatory mechanisms are referred to as *cardiac reserve*. The patient who has congestive heart failure and whose heart has compensated by dilatation, has already used up much of his or her cardiac reserve and can no longer respond as well to stress (Figure 6.1b).

In summary, heart failure is manifested by reduced cardiac output, increased sympathetic tone of blood vessels (which puts even more pressure on the left ventricle), fluid retention, increased intravascular volume, edema of the lungs and lower extremities, myocardial dilatation, and loss of cardiac reserve.

DRUGS USED FOR TREATING HEART FAILURE

The classic drugs used to treat congestive heart failure are glycosides obtained from the leaves of the foxglove, *Digitalis purpurea*; from a related plant, *Digitalis lanata*; and from *Strophantus gratus*.

FIGURE 6.1

Frank-Starling response to stretching of cardiac muscle fibers in a normal heart (*a*) and a failing heart (*b*). Note the reduction in cardiac reserve as indicated by a reduced cardiac output with exertion.

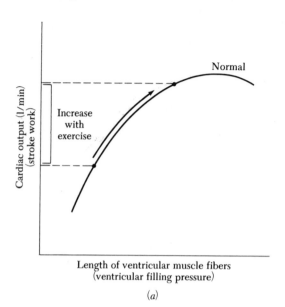

(*a*)

(*b*)

DRUGS USED FOR CARDIAC AND VASCULAR DISORDERS

TABLE 6.1
Sources of commonly used cardiac glycosides

Digitalis purpurea	*Digitalis lanata*	*Strophanthus gratus*
Digitoxin	Digoxin	Ouabain
Digoxin	Lanatoside C	
Digitalis leaf	Deslanoside	

They also are obtained from squill (the dried bulb of the sea onion), *Convallaria majalis* (lily of the valley), *Thevetia neriifolia* (yellow oleander), and the dried skin of the common toad. The alkaloids obtained from *Digitalis* and *Strophanthus* are listed in Table 6.1. More recently, a new class of drugs called the bipyridines, of which amrinone (Inocor) is the prototype, has been introduced.

DIGITALIS

The term digitalis applies to the dried leaf of the common foxglove. While occasionally still used, digitalis itself essentially has been replaced by *digoxin* (Lanoxin), a purified alkaloid from *Digitalis lanata*. The following discussion will refer to digoxin but what is said about this compound applies equally to all glycosides of digitalis.

The chemical structure of digoxin is shown in Figure 6.2. As illustrated, this *cardiac glycoside* is made up of a steroid moiety and three molecules of sugar (digitoxoses). The pharmacologic activity resides in the steroid portion, but the particular sugars modify the solubility and cell penetrability of the various glycosides.

EFFECT OF CARDIAC GLYCOSIDES ON THE FAILING HEART

Digoxin and the other cardiac glycosides increase the contractility of the heart muscle, thereby increasing cardiac reserves (Figure 6.3). This positive inotropic effect occurs in both the normal and the failing heart. The increased force of contraction results in more complete emptying of the ventricles and thus a reduction in the physical size of the failing heart. As a result, tension in myocardial fibers is decreased, and both the energy requirements and the rate of oxygen consumption of the heart cells are reduced. In other

FIGURE 6.2
Effect of digoxin on the failing heart. (Compare with Figure 6.1*b*.)

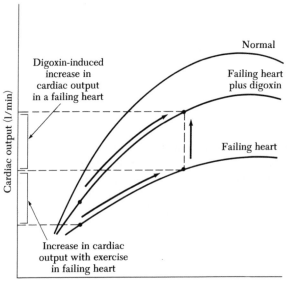

Length of ventricular muscle fibers

words, the resulting increased efficiency of myocardial contraction is responsible for increased cardiac output, decreased heart size, increased ventricular emptying, and increased cardiac reserve.

The mechanism of action of digitalis appears to involve inhibition of the enzyme sodium-potassium-activated adenosine triphosphatase, which leads to an increase in intracellular calcium concentrations. This enzyme is involved in the active transport of sodium and potassium ions across cardiac cell membranes. Its inhibition leads to an increase in intracellular sodium and a decrease in intracellular potassium. An increase in intracellular sodium is crucial since intracellular calcium normally is exchanged for extracellular sodium along gradient-dependent transport systems. When intracellular sodium is increased as a result of digoxin-induced ATPase inhibition, the exchange of extracellular sodium for intracellular calcium is diminished and the concentration of intracellular calcium increases. This process most likely leads to increased stores of calcium in the muscle fibers; at each electrical impulse the greater quantities of calcium released augment contraction of myocardial muscle fibers.

FIGURE 6.3
Structure of digoxin (Lanoxin), the most widely used cardiac glycoside.

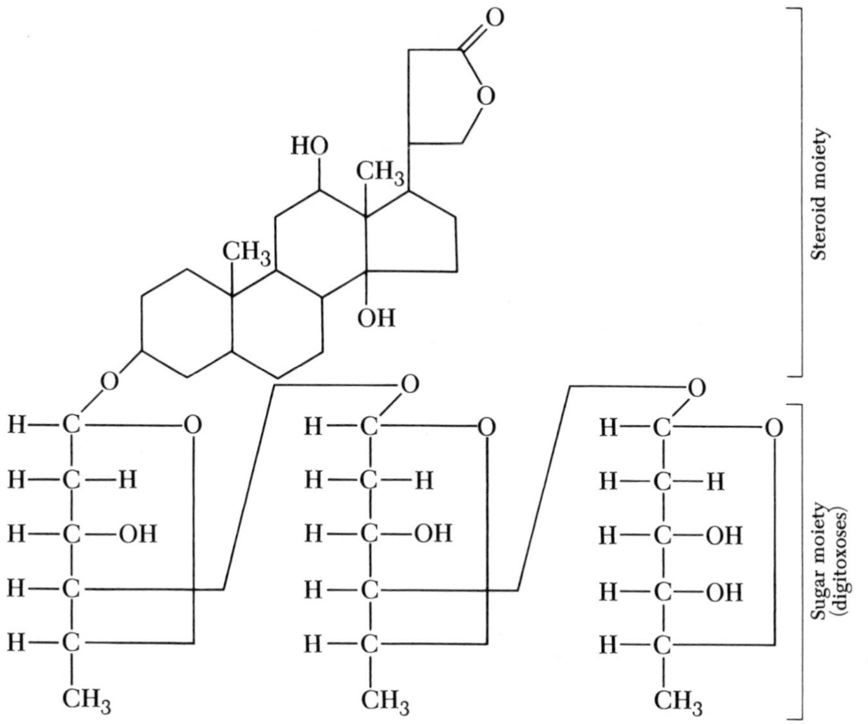

EFFECTS OF CARDIAC GLYCOSIDES ON THE ELECTROPHYSIOLOGY OF THE HEART

Digoxin and the other cardiac glycosides have important therapeutic and toxic effects on the electrophysiologic properties of the conducting system of the heart. Although these effects are complex, they can be briefly outlined as follows. Digoxin slows conduction of electrical impulses through the AV node, which reduces the numbers of atrial impulses that can be conducted through the node to the ventricles. As a result, digoxin is useful clinically as an antiarrhythmic agent in the treatment of atrial flutter and atrial fibrillation. Digoxin does not stop the atrial flutter or fibrillation but only slows the ventricular rate associated with it. Other electrophysiologic effects of the cardiac glycosides on the heart are very complicated and may be found in the classic textbooks of pharmacology.

EFFECTS OF DIGOXIN OUTSIDE THE HEART

At therapeutic doses, digoxin and the other cardiac glycosides primarily affect the heart. As blood levels of the drug increase (see below), however, significant systemic effects may be observed. Gastrointestinal effects are manifested as nausea and loss of appetite. Neurologic symptoms may include altered vision and a toxic psychosis. The diuretic effect reflects the increased cardiac output, improved circulation, and decreased aldosterone release (Chapter 11) and is considered to be part of the therapeutic effect of digoxin in relieving fluid retention and edema.

DIGOXIN TOXICITY

Digoxin toxicity, and that of other cardiac glycosides, is common. The therapeutic range of these drugs is very narrow [for digoxin 1 to 2 nanograms per milliliter (ng/ml)]. Levels below approximately 1 ng/ml are subtherapeutic, and levels above approximately 2 ng/ml produce increasing toxicity. Symptoms of mild toxicity may include vomiting, loss of appetite, bradycardia, visual disturbances, and mild cardiac arrhythmias. More severe toxicity results in an increased incidence of virtually every type of cardiac arrhythmia, the most dangerous being ventricular in origin because it can lead to ventricular fibrillation and death. Elderly patients and patients taking diuretics, which cause potassium loss, are especially prone to digitalis intoxication. Drug interactions with digoxin are extremely common. All patients taking a cardiac glycoside should be closely monitored, and no additional medications should be taken without the advice of a physician.

CLINICAL USES OF DIGOXIN

Digoxin currently is the drug of choice for the treatment of congestive heart failure and for slowing the ventricular rate in patients with atrial flutter and atrial fibrillation.

ALTERNATIVES TO DIGOXIN

Although digoxin and other cardiac glycosides improve cardiac contractility, peripheral vascular resistance often remains high and organ perfusion only marginally improves. What is often needed, therefore, is a combination of the positive inotropic effect induced by digoxin and a reduction in peripheral vascular resistance, such as that achieved by vasodilatation. (Vasodilators are discussed in Chapter 9.)

Continuing research has sought to develop new agents that combine positive inotropy with peripheral vasodilatation. The intravenous form of one of these drugs, amrinone, has recently been approved and marketed for the treatment of severe congestive heart failure in hospitalized patients. Amrinone increases myocardial contractility and causes smooth muscle relaxation, therefore, improving cardiac output and reducing systemic vascular resistance. Its mechanism of action involves inhibition of the enzyme phosphodiesterase; this produces increased levels of cyclic adenosine monophosphate and, as a result, mediates increased cardiac contractility and peripheral vasodilatation.

Limitations to amrinone include its availability only in intravenous form and a high incidence of possibly serious side effects, including reductions in platelet count (thrombocytopenia) and liver toxicity. Other derivatives of amrinone (e.g., milrinone) are under evaluation in attempts to minimize the side effects and provide an alternative to digoxin therapy.

R E A D I N G S

American Medical Association, "Agents Uses to Treat Heart Failure," in *AMA Drug Evaluations*, 6th ed., American Medical Association, Chicago, 1986, pp. 419–434.

Braunwald, E. (ed.), "A Symposium: Amrinone," *Amer. J. Cardiology*, **56**:1B–42B (1985).

Cowan, F. F., *Pharmacology for the Dental Hygienist*, Lea & Febiger, Philadelphia, 1978, pp. 306–343.

Hoffman, B. F., and J. T. Bigger, "Digitalis and Allied Cardiac Glycosides," in A. G. Gilman, L. S. Goodman, T. W. Rall, and F. Murad (eds.), *The Pharmacological Basis of Therapeutics*, 7th ed., Macmillan, New York, 1985, pp. 716–747.

CHAPTER 7

DRUG TREATMENT
OF CARDIAC ARRHYTHMIAS

OVERVIEW OF CARDIAC ARRHYTHMIAS

Antiarrhythmic drugs are useful both in the acute treatment and in the long-term prevention of disorders of cardiac rhythm. Cardiac arrhythmias may be relatively benign in patients who can maintain normal cardiac output, or they may be associated with very high rates of fatality. Cardiac arrhythmias arise from abnormal rates of impulse generation in the SA node, from abnormal (ectopic) sites of impulse initiation, and from disturbances in the conduction of electrical impulses (Table 7.1).

TABLE 7.1
Types and causes of cardiac arrhythmias

Type	Cause
Sinus arrhythmia	
Sinus bradycardia	Athletic training
	Sinus dysfunction
Sinus tachycardia	Increased sympathetic tone
	Increased thyroid function
	Fever
	Heart failure
Sick sinus syndrome	SA node block
	Sinus node disorders
Atrial (non–SA node) arrhythmias	
Premature atrial contractions	Excessive caffeine, nicotine, and alcohol
	Heart failure
Paroxysmal atrial tachycardia	Increased catecholamine levels or sensitivity
	Digitalis toxicity
	Conduction block with "re-entry"
Nodal rhythm	SA node depression (e.g., by increased vagal activity)
Atrial flutter	⎧ Damage to atrial muscle
Atrial fibrilation	⎨ Cardiomyopathy
	⎩ Re-entry (circus movement)
Ventricular arrhythmias	
Premature ventricular contractions	Ischemic heart disease
	Prior myocardial infarction
	Digitalis toxicity
	Increased catecholamine sensitivity
Ventricular tachycardia	Cardiomyopathies
Ventricular flutter	Cardiomyopathies
Ventricular fibrillation	Cardiomyopathies

SINUS ARRHYTHMIAS

As presented in Chapter 5, the SA node usually functions as the pacemaker for initiation of the cardiac electrical impulse. The normal sinus rate ranges from about 55 to 100 beats per minute and is regular in rhythm because the time period between each beat is constant. Irregularities in rhythm or rates outside the normal range technically are classified as arrhythmias. *Sinus bradycardia* refers to a regular rhythm with a rate below 55 beats per minute, and *sinus tachycardia* refers to a regular rhythm with a rate above 100 beats per minute. Patients with irregular sinus rhythms because of SA node dysfunction are considered to have a *sick sinus syndrome.*

Sinus bradycardia does not require treatment if cardiac output is normal. Trained athletes, for example, often have rates below 50 beats per minute at rest and can greatly increase their cardiac output with only modest increases above this. If bradycardia results in failure to supply sufficient cardiac output to meet body demands, atropine (Chapter 3) may increase the sinus rate temporarily; for permanent relief an implanted battery-operated pacemaker may be needed.

Sinus tachycardia can result from increased activity of the sympathetic nervous system, from increases in thyroid gland activity, from fever, and even from congestive heart failure. If tachycardia persists after treatment of these underlying causes, a beta blocking drug (Chapter 3 and pp. 73–74) may be useful.

Patients with sick sinus syndrome seldom respond to drug treatment. Permanent pacemakers usually are required to prevent the hypotension and fainting episodes that accompany the bradycardia associated with the syndrome.

ATRIAL ARRHYTHMIAS

Non-SA node arrhythmias arising in ectopic foci of the atria include premature atrial contractions (PAC), paroxysmal atrial tachycardia (PAT), nodal rhythm (arising in the AV node), atrial flutter, and atrial fibrillation. PAC or nodal rhythm usually is innocuous, often requires no pharmacologic treatment, and usually responds to the elimination of their principal cause, such as the excessive use of caffeine, nicotine, or alcohol. Control of congestive heart failure with digoxin generally controls the PAC associated with this disorder.

PAT refers to the rapid heart rate in which the impulse originates in the atria, outside the AV node. PAT is thought to be caused by "reentry" mechanisms or self-supporting "circus movement" of impulses around the atrial muscle. Numerous drugs have been used in the treatment of PAT, and these are discussed below. Currently, the calcium channel blockers such as *verapamil* are playing an increased role as first-line treatment of persistent PAT.

Atrial flutter and atrial fibrillation refer to extremely rapid rates of atrial activity (usually with equally rapid rates of ventricular activity) unless AV nodal conduction is reduced. The atrial rate during atrial flutter usually is 250 to 350 beats per minute and quite regular. The atrial rate during atrial fibrillation, on the other hand, usually is 350 to 600 beats per minute, totally disorganized, and without effective atrial contraction. Such rapid rates of activity seldom allow sufficient time for ventricular filling or emptying and result in reduced cardiac output. Thus, the primary goal in treating atrial flutter and atrial fibrillation is to reduce the ventricular rate to near-normal levels, while the secondary goal is to restore a normal sinus rhythm. A variety of pharmacological and nonpharmacologic interventions are available. Clinically, digoxin often is preferred because of its ability to decrease the conduction of impulses through the AV node. More recently, however, verapamil has been used both because of its digoxinlike action on the AV node and because it may convert the atrial flutter to normal sinus rhythm. Electrical cardioversion also is effective in terminating atrial flutter and atrial fibrillation and restoring normal sinus rhythm. Quinidine, along with digoxin, is used for long-term therapy to prevent recurrence of atrial flutter and atrial fibrillation.

VENTRICULAR ARRHYTHMIAS

Ventricular arrhythmias include occasional premature ventricular contractions (PVC), ventricular tachycardia, ventricular flutter, and ventricular fibrillation. Occasional PVCs in patients without coronary artery disease or underlying heart disease usually are of little clinical significance and generally do not require treatment. Frequent PVCs, however, are associated with an increased risk of sudden death due to their progression to more serious ventricular arrhythmias. Ventricular tachycardia is a serious disorder because it may lead to reductions in cardiac output, decreased coronary artery perfusion, ventricular fibrillation, and death. Antiarrhythmic drugs are used to treat persistent episodes of ventricular tachycardia and to prevent their reoccurrence. Agents used to treat rapid onset, life-threatening ventricular tachycardia include lidocaine, procainamide, and bretylium. Several drugs used for long-term suppression of serious ventricular arrhythmias include quinidine, procainamide, and beta blocking agents, such as propranolol.

MISCELLANEOUS ARRHYTHMIAS

While digoxin is used as an antiarrhythmic drug to decrease ventricular rate in atrial flutter and atrial fibrillation, digitalis toxicity can cause virtually any cardiac arrhythmia, especially atrial and ventricular premature contractions (PAC and PVC) and tachycardias (PAT and PVT). The mechanism involves a digoxin-induced decrease in the refractory period of atrial and ventricular muscle fibers, predisposing them to rapid rates of discharge. Lidocaine and phenytoin (Dilantin) are drugs of choice for treating digoxin-induced arrhythmias, although other more sophisticated interventions may be necessary.

PHARMACOLOGY OF ANTIARRHYTHMIC DRUGS

Antiarrhythmic drugs can be conveniently classified into five groups. These are presented in Table 7.2.

CARDIAC DEPRESSANTS

The cardiac depressants are general depressants of myocardial electrical activity; they increase the refractory period of heart muscle, thereby abolishing reentry arrhythmias. They also decrease the excitability of heart muscle, decrease ectopic activity, and decrease myocardial contractility.

Quinidine

Quinidine is closely related to quinine, a drug used for the treatment of malaria. Both drugs are found as alkaloids in cinchona, the bark of the South American cinchona tree. Quinidine depresses the spontaneous rate of depolarization of myocardial cells and increases the refractory period. This general cardiac depressant is useful in treating atrial and ventricular premature contractions and atrial and ventricular tachycardias (Table 7.3). It is used primarily to maintain normal sinus rhythm after electrical cardioversion of atrial flutter or atrial fibrillation and to prevent premature ventricular contractions and ventricular tachycardia. It is well absorbed orally, is highly bound to plasma proteins, is largely metabolized in the liver, and is partially excreted by the kidneys. Its half-life is about 6 hours. The drug is usually given orally, since parenteral injection can be dangerous. Nausea, vomiting, and diarrhea are common side effects. Other, more serious side effects include ECG changes, hypotension, cinchonism (ringing in the ears, blurred vision, seeing flashes of light, confusion, and psychosis), and allergic responses. Quinidine is available under multiple trade names including Quinidex, Quinaglute, and Cardioquin.

TABLE 7.2
Classes of antiarrhythmic drugs

Cardiac depressants	Primary uses	Electrophysiologic actions
Quinidine Procainamide Disopyramide	Atrial and ventricular arrhythmias, chronic	Increased refractory period
Lidocaine Phenytoin	Acute, ventricular arrhythmias Digoxin-induced ventricular arrhythmias	Decreased spontaneous depolarization
Beta-adrenergic blockers		
Propranolol	Atrial tachycardia	Reduced catecholamine sensitivity Reduced heart rate Reduced conduction velocity Decreased contractility
Cardiac glycosides		
Digoxin	Atrial flutter and fibrillation	Reduced conduction through AV node Decreased ventricular refractory period
Calcium channel blockers		
Verapamil	Atrial flutter and fibrillation Paroxysmal atrial tachycardia	Reduced SA node depolarization Decreased contractility Reduced AV node conduction Increased refractory period of myocardium
Adrenergic blocking agent		
Bretylium	Severe ventricular arrhythmias	Decreased norepinephrine release Increased refractory period of myocardium

Procainamide (Pronestyl)

Closely resembling quinidine in its actions is procainamide (see Figure 7.1). Its clinical uses in relieving atrial and ventricular arrhythmias are nearly identical to those of quinidine. It is well absorbed orally, is only slightly bound to plasma proteins, is excreted largely unchanged by the kidneys, and has a half-life of only about 3 hours. Nausea, vomiting, and diarrhea occur less often than with quinidine, but about 30 percent of patients taking procainamide for

TABLE 7.3
Relative utility of antiarrhythmic drugs in the treatment of specific cardiac arrhythmias*

Arrhythmia	Quinidine	Procainamide	Disopyramide	Lidocaine	Phenytoin	Propranolol	Bretylium	Verapamil
Atrial								
Atrial fibrillation, conversion	2	2	1	0	0	1	0	1
Atrial fibrillation, prophylaxis	3	3	3	0	0	2	0	2
Atrial fibrillation, rate control	0	0	0	0	0	2	0	3
Atrial premature contractions	2	2	2	0	1	3	0	4
Ventricular								
Ventricular premature contractions	3	3	3	4	2	1	1	1
Ventricular tachycardia	3	3	2	3	2	1	2	1
Digitalis-induced arrhythmias	1	1	1	3	3	2	0	0

* The relative utility score is based on an overall estimate of efficacy, convenience, and toxicity. The scale of relative utility is as follows: 0, none; 1, poor; 2, fair; 3, good; 4, excellent.

SOURCE: Modified from J. T. Bigger and B. F. Hoffman, "Antiarrhythmic Drugs," in A. G. Gilman, L. S. Goodman, T. W. Rall, and F. Murad (eds.), *The Pharmacological Basis of Therapeutics*, 7th ed., Macmillan, New York, 1985, p. 757.

prolonged periods develop hypersensitivity to the drug. Fevers, arthralgias, blood cell reactions, and other serious problems can result from such hypersensitivity. Thus, the risks of taking the drug must be weighed against the protection it affords against serious cardiac arrhythmias.

Disopyramide (Norpace)
Disopyramide's action is similar to that of quinidine and procainamide. It is used occasionally for serious ventricular arrhythmias in adults, although anticholinergic side effects are significant. Because it can cause some adverse effects on blood pressure, its use is limited, especially in patients with heart failure.

Lidocaine (Xylocaine)
The widely used local anesthetic lidocaine also is extremely effective intravenously as an antiarrhythmic agent against serious ventricular arrhythmias of sudden onset, especially in patients who have just experienced a myocardial infarction. Indeed, for such patients it may be lifesaving. It also is widely used prophylactically in hospitalized patients who have had a recent myocardial infarction to protect them against the sudden onset of ventricular arrhythmias.

Phenytoin (Dilantin)
Phenytoin is an antiepileptic drug with antiarrhythmic properties. It depresses spontaneous depolarization of ventricular cells and is used primarily to treat the ventricular arrhythmias associated with digoxin overdosage. Absorption is erratic after oral administration and the drug is metabolized before it is excreted. Its half-life is about 18 hours and it is highly bound to plasma proteins. Numerous side effects are seen with the drug but usually these are well-tolerated. Therapeutic blood levels are in the range of 10 to 20 micrograms per kilogram (μg/kg).

BETA-ADRENERGIC BLOCKING DRUGS

Several drugs classified as beta-adrenergic blocking agents (Chapter 3) are used as antiarrhythmic agents, in addition to their being used effectively as antihypertensive and antianginal agents (Chapter 8). While not frequently used as antiarrhythmics, beta blockers such as *propranolol* (*Inderal*) reduce the responsiveness of the AV node and the myocardium to endogenous catecholamines; they also decrease heart rate, slow conduction of electrical impulses to the AV node, and decreases contractility. Because of these actions, propranolol is used primarily to treat atrial tachycardias such as PAT, atrial flutter, and atrial fibrillation. Propranolol's side effects are related to the beta blockade. Because the heart usually compensates for its reduced performance during heart failure by increasing sympathetic tone (Chapter 6), beta blockade may lead to hypotension and aggravation of the heart failure. Pulmonary side effects include precipitation of bronchospasm. The treatment of hypertension with propranolol is discussed in Chapter 9.

CARDIAC GLYCOSIDES

As stated above, the cardiac glycosides including *digoxin* are an important class of antiarrhythmic drugs, especially in the treatment of atrial flutter and atrial fibrillation, because they decrease the ventricular rate without affecting the flutter or fibrillation. Sinus tachycardia and PAT associated with congestive heart failure also may respond to digoxin therapy. Digoxin's ability to shorten the ventricular refractory period, and thus increase cellular excitability, increases the susceptibility to ventricular arrhythmias, especially as blood levels rise above the therapeutic range (see Chapter 6). Thus, digoxin acts both as an arrhythmogenic and as an antiarrhythmic.

CALCIUM CHANNEL BLOCKERS

The calcium channel blockers, especially *verapamil (Calan)*, are being used increasingly as antiarrhythmic agents. As discussed in Chapter 5, the inward movement of calcium ions through "slow calcium channels" is involved in the genesis of the depolarization of cardiac cells and therefore in the generation of the cardiac electrical impulse. Inward calcium movement is also involved in the contraction of the cardiac muscle fibers and in energy storage and utilization. Drug-induced blockade of calcium channels, therefore, would be expected to reduce both the generation of cardiac impulses and the contractility of cardiac muscle. Such drugs depress cardiac excitability and contractility, and, as such, they are useful as antiarrhythmic agents. Calcium channel blockers also produce dilatation of blood vessels, making them clinically useful as antianginal drugs (Chapter 8).

In the heart, the pacemaker cells of the SA node and certain cells in the region of the AV node are dependent on the inward movement of calcium through these calcium channels. Thus, the calcium channel blockers (especially verapamil) depress the rate of SA node depolarization, reduce the conduction of impulses through the AV node, prolong the refractory period of myocardial cells, and depress myocardial contractility. These drugs help control atrial arrhythmias, both those of the reentry type (atrial flutter and fibrillation) and PAT. Indeed, verapamil often will convert PAT to a normal sinus rhythm. Long-term oral therapy with verapamil appears to decrease the frequency, duration, and severity of atrial arrhythmias. Clinically this is often manifested as increased exercise tolerance and decreased palpitations during exertion.

BRETYLIUM

Bretylium (Bretylol) is a parenterally administered drug that decreases the release of norepinephrine from sympathetic nerve terminals and directly prolongs the refractory period of myocardial cells. It is used in the treatment of severe ventricular arrhythmias, especially those seen in cardial arrests, that fail to respond to other, more traditional antiarrhythmics such as lidocaine and cardioversion. Bretylium may facilitate successful electrical cardioversion of arrhythmias where prior attempts at cardioversion were unsuccessful. Its effects are slow in onset after intravenous injection, requiring up to 20 or 30 minutes. The drug is excreted unchanged by the kidneys and has a half-life of about 8 to 12 hours. Initial hypertension, caused by an initial NE release, is followed by prolonged hypotension. There are numerous other side effects but usually these are of secondary concern relative to the lifethreatening circumstances under which bretylium is used.

READINGS

American Medical Association, "Antiarrhythmic Drugs," in *AMA Drug Evaluations*, 6th ed., American Medical Association, Chicago, 1986, pp. 435–461.

Bigger, J. T., and B. F. Hoffman, "Antiarrhythmic Drugs," in A. G. Gilman, L. S. Goodman, and A. Gilman (eds.), *The Pharmacological Basis of Therapeutics*, 7th ed., Macmillan, New York, 1985, pp. 748–783.

Luderer, J., "Antiarrhythmic Drugs," in A. Goth (ed.), *Medical Pharmacology*, Mosby, St. Louis, 1984, pp. 436–451.

CHAPTER 8

DRUG TREATMENT
OF ANGINA PECTORIS

Angina pectoris, the principal symptom of ischemic heart disease, is manifested by sudden, severe, pressing chest pain that often radiates to the left shoulder and down the left arm. Attacks of "classic" angina are the result of temporary ischemia of heart muscle; that is, the flow of blood through the coronary arteries to the heart muscle does not meet the oxygen requirements of the heart muscle, especially when exertion increases oxygen demand. In "variant" angina, spasm of the coronary arteries occurs at rest and oxygen deficits occur secondary to this spasm and are not necessarily a result of increased oxygen requirements. The chest pain caused by

FIGURE 8.1
Structures of representative antianginal drugs.

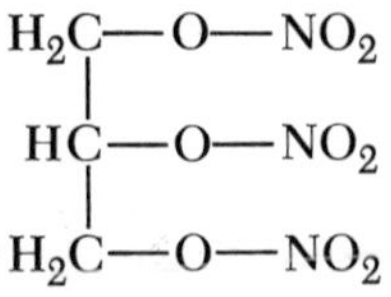

Nitroglycerine
(glyceryl trinitrate)

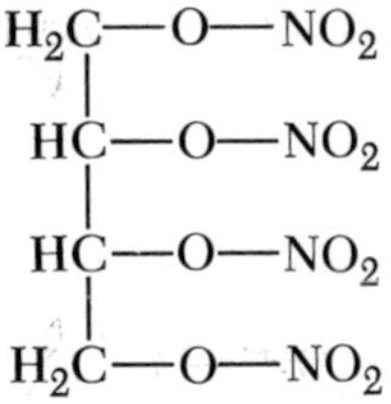

Erythrityl tetranitrate

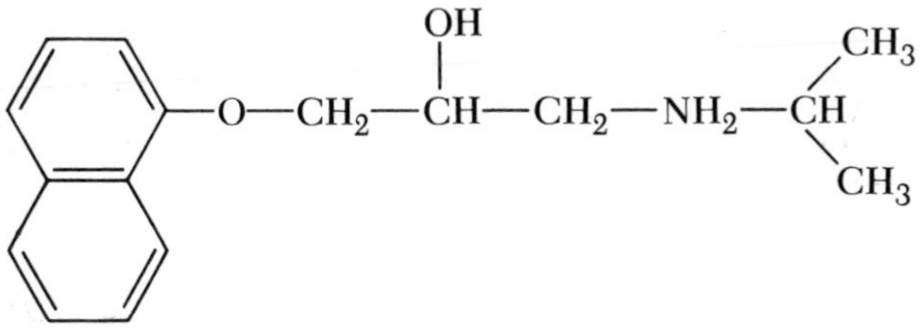

Propranolol

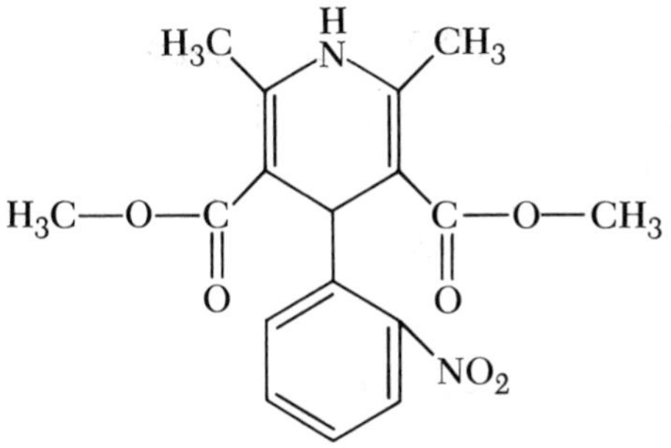

Nifedipine

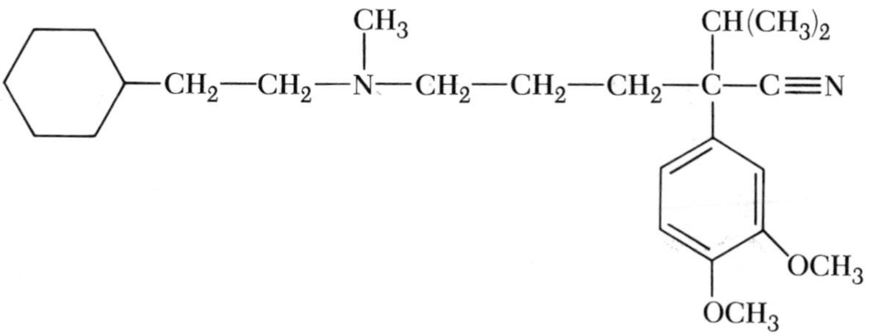

Verapamil

both types of angina is relieved quickly by nitroglycerin (Figure 8.1). Although nitroglycerin and other drugs also may afford more long-term relief, they do not correct the underlying causes of reduced coronary artery blood flow.

Treatment with antianginal drugs is only part of a general program to alleviate symptoms and reduce risk factors that predispose to coronary artery disease. Cessation of smoking is essential, and in obese patients, weight loss may produce improvement. Dietary modifications, especially efforts to reduce blood cholesterol levels, may be advantageous. Control of hypertension (Chapter 9) leads to a decrease in myocardial work and therefore to decreased myocardial oxygen demands. This alone may relieve angina. Young adults with a family history of coronary artery disease and "heart problems" would be wise to reduce their risk factors long before the symptoms of angina indicate the presence of coronary artery disease.

PHARMACOLOGIC MANAGEMENT OF ANGINA PECTORIS

The drugs used to treat angina pectoris are listed in Table 8.1. In acute situations, the sublingual (under-the-tongue) use of nitroglycerin will prevent or relieve an attack. For long-term protection, the beta-adrenergic blocking agents, oral and topical nitrates, and the calcium channel blockers are all effective. The mechanisms through which each of these works are different, which necessitates separate discussion and allowing for combined use in cases where symptoms are difficult to control.

NITROGLYCERIN

Nitroglycerin is a liquid that is adsorbed to a tablet for convenience of sublingual administration. It is the drug of choice for treatment of acute anginal attacks. In unopened, darkened glass bottles, its shelf-life is about 6 months; when the bottle is opened, the medication deteriorates within a few weeks. Onset of activity with sublingual use occurs within 1 to 3 minutes and effects last about 10 to 20 minutes. Early attempts to explain nitroglycerin's action focused on its vasodilating properties, and concluded that nitroglycerin improved blood flow to ischemic areas of the heart by dilating coronary arteries. The current point of view is that nitroglycerin

TABLE 8.1
Drugs for angina pectoris

Drug	Route of administration	Mechanism of action
	Nitroglycerine	
Nitroglycerine	Sublingual Topical Buccal Intravenous Transdermal	Venodilatation (reduced "preload") Modest reduction in peripheral vascular resistance ("afterload") Mild dilatation of coronary arteries
	Oral nitrates	
Isosorbide dinitrate	Oral, sublingual	Same as nitroglycerine
Erythrityl tetranitrate	Oral	
Pentaerythritol tetranitrate	Oral	
	Beta-adrenergic blockers	
Propranolol	Oral, intravenous	Beta blockade Decreased heart rate Decreased force of contraction
Atenolol	Oral	
Metoprolol	Oral	
Nadolol	Oral	
Timolol	Oral	
Acebutolol	Oral	
Labetalol	Oral, intravenous	
	Calcium channel blockers	
Verapamil	Oral, intravenous	Calcium channel blockade Coronary artery dilitation Relief of coronary artery spasm
Nifedipine	Oral	Reduced afterload
Diltiazem	Oral	Cardiac depression

reduces myocardial oxygen requirements through its actions on the systemic circulation. Nitroglycerin's reduction of venous tone (dilation of the veins) results in a pooling of blood in the peripheral veins. Nitroglycerin also reduces return of blood to the heart, which reduces the volume of blood in the ventricle and thus decreases the tension on the walls of the ventricles. Its ability to decrease peripheral vascular resistance reduces arterial blood pressure, thereby decreasing the resistance against which the left ventricle must pump. A degree of coronary artery dilatation may also be involved. Thus, nitroglycerin may be thought of primarily as a *venodilator* with a modest degree of arterial vasodilatation and a very mild degree of coronary artery vasodilatation.

Nitroglycerin is available in tablets for sublingual use, as a liquid for intravenous infusion, in ointments for topical use, and in transdermal "patches" that release the drug continuously through the skin over a 24-hour period.

ORAL NITRATES

Efforts to extend nitroglycerin's duration of action lead to the development of the *oral nitrates*. These drugs include isosorbide dinitrate (Isordil, Sorbitrate), erythrityl tetranitrate (Cardilate), and pentaerythritol tetranitrate (Peritrate). The oral compounds have a longer duration of action than sublingual preparations and when used for long-term prevention of classic angina, can improve exercise tolerance and reduce the need for sublingual nitroglycerin. They are well absorbed from the stomach, but because they are quite rapidly metabolized by the liver, rather large doses may be required to achieve therapeutic effects. Side effects encountered with these agents, and with nitroglycerin, include headaches, flushing, dizziness, hypotension, and reflex tachycardia—all of which can be explained by the vasodilatation produced. Tolerance and dependence develop to a significant degree and are more prevalent in patients on long-term therapy with orally administered preparations.

BETA-ADRENERGIC BLOCKERS

The beta-adrenergic blockers are widely used in the treatment of classical angina pectoris. Their effectiveness is due to their ability to reduce both heart rate and the force of contraction, thus reducing the oxygen demands of the heart. Available beta blockers include propranolol (Inderal), metoprolol (Lopressor), labetalol (Trandate), acebutolol (Sectral), atenolol (Tenormin), and nadolol (Corgard). Of these, metoprolol and atenolol appear to be the most cardioselective since they have relatively greater $beta_1$ blocking activity and relatively less $beta_2$ blocking ability. Even with these, however, the relief of symptoms of angina must be balanced carefully against the possible detrimental effects on cardiac function in patients with borderline cardiac reserves who rely on sympathetic stimulation to maintain a level of activity.

In general, however, the beta-adrenergic blockers are important in the long-term management of angina pectoris, significantly reducing the amount of nitroglycerin patients must consume. Because these agents and nitroglycerin reduce cardiac work by different mechanisms, they have a synergistic effect on the heart in reducing its oxygen requirements. Because the beta blockers also reduce heart rate and contraction force, they tend to prevent or reduce the reflex tachycardia that follows the vasodilatation and the fall in blood pressure induced by nitroglycerin. Heart rate is commonly monitored as an index of the activity of these drugs. Careful monitoring for heart failure in susceptible patients is strongly advised as well.

CALCIUM CHANNEL BLOCKERS

As discussed in Chapter 7, the cardiac depressant effects of the calcium channel blockers make them useful antiarrhythmic agents. In addition, calcium movement across cellular membranes controls vascular tone in the smooth muscle of both the coronary and the peripheral blood vessels. Such calcium movement may be blocked by the calcium channel blockers. Verapamil (Calan), nifedipine (Procardia), and diltiazem (Cardizem) are the three calcium channel blockers currently available. Of these three, nifedipine and diltiazem appear to have a relatively greater effect on reducing the tone of vascular smooth muscle and less effect on cardiac muscle. They also are most effective at producing calcium channel blockade, which results in increased blood flow through coronary arteries. Clinically, these drugs appear to be most effective against variant angina, the type most refractory to long-term beta blocker therapy. Their interference with calcium entry into vascular smooth muscle results in coronary vasodilatation, relief of coronary artery spasm, and reduction in peripheral vascular resistance—all of which are beneficial to the patient.

Nifedipine is effective against and reduces the frequency of variant angina attacks, which are refractory to oral nitrates and beta blockers, decreases nitroglycerin requirements, and improves exercise tolerance. It exerts little depressant effect on the heart and does not precipitate bronchospasm. Major side effects include the risk of significant episodes of hypotension.

Diltiazem possesses both cardiac depressant and vasodilator actions. The drug is therefore effective in reducing myocardial oxygen requirements and increasing myocardial oxygen supply—a most beneficial effect. Thus, it reduces the frequency of anginal attacks and decreases nitroglycerin requirements. As expected, side effects reflecting the cardiac depression and the peripheral vasodilatation are prominent.

In summary, the four classes of drugs discussed—nitroglycerin, oral nitrates, beta-adrenergic blockers, and calcium channel blockers—all contribute to a beneficial supply and demand ratio either by reducing myocardial work or by increasing myocardial oxygen supply. Nitroglycerin remains the first drug of choice for acute attacks and the other three classes of agents are added as tolerated to reduce nitroglycerin requirements, reduce the severity of anginal attacks, and improve exercise tolerance. Once again, close physician guidance is imperative and patient education regarding the goals and limitations of therapy, as well as a reduction in risk factors, must be an important part of the overall therapeutic plan.

R E A D I N G S

Abrams, J., "Pharmacology of Nitroglycerin and Long-Acting Nitrates," *Amer. J. Cardiology*, **56**:12A–18A (1985).

American Medical Association, "Antianginal Agents," in *AMA Drug Evaluations*, 6th ed., American Medical Association, Chicago, 1986, pp. 463–481.

Conti, C. R., C. J. Pepine, R. L. Feldman, and J. A. Hill, "Calcium Antagonists," *Cardiology*, **72**:297–321 (1985).

Corwin, S., and J. A. Reiffel, "Nitrate Therapy for Angina Pectoris. Current Concepts about Mechanism of Action and Evaluation of Currently Available Preparations," *Arch. Intern. Med.*, **145**:538–543 (1985).

Johns, V. J., "Beta-blocking Drugs for Arrhythmias, Hypertension, and Ischemic Heart Disease," *Amer. J. Surgery*, **147**:725–730 (1984).

Leon, M. B., et al., "Combination Therapy with Calcium Channel Blockers and Beta Blockers for Chronic Stable Angina Pectoris," *Amer. J. Cardiology*, **55**:69B–80B (1985).

Needleman, P., P. B. Corr, and E. M. Johnson, "Drugs Used for the Treatment of Angina," in A. G. Gilman, L. S. Goodman, T. W. Rall, and F. Murad (eds.), *The Pharmacological Basis of Therapeutics*, 7th ed., Macmillan, New York, 1985, pp. 806–826.

Sorkin, E. M., S. P. Clissold, and R. N. Brogden, "Nifedipine. A Review of its Pharmacodynamic and Pharmacokinetic Properties and Therapeutic Efficacy in Ischemic Heart Disease, Hypertension, and Related Cardiovascular Disorders," *Drugs*, **30**(3):182–274 (1985).

Syposium, "Ischemic Heart Disease: The Role of Isordil—Past, Present, and Future," *Amer. Heart J.*, **1**(2):197–292 (1985).

ANTIHYPERTENSIVE DRUGS

Hypertension is one of the significant risk factors in the long-term development of such serious cardiovascular disorders as congestive heart failure, coronary artery disease, heart attack, stroke, and kidney failure. Hypertension contributes mightily to premature death and disability. Excessive sodium chloride (salt) intake and obesity both appear to play an important role in the genesis of "essential hypertension" (i.e., that which cannot be ascribed to specific causes such as narrowing of the renal artery, tumors of the adrenal glands, and so forth). Weight control, reduction of salt intake, and pharmacologic treatment are the mainstays of the current hypertension therapy. Hypertensive patients may improve the quality and length of their lives by achieving strict control of blood pressure, maintaining ideal body weight, reducing salt intake, adhering to pharmacologic recommendations, and controlling other risk factors associated with cardiovascular disease, such as stopping smoking, lowering blood cholesterol, and increasing physical conditioning. The present discussion will focus on the pharmacologic treatment of hypertension, although other lifestyle alterations are of equal importance.

Should all cases of hypertension be treated? Here, the answer is a qualified yes! First, one must know his or her own resting blood pressure. An ideal blood pressure might be 120/80 mmHg, with 120 mmHg being the systolic pressure achieved during the period of cardiac contraction and 80 mmHg the diastolic pressure achieved during cardiac filling. A diastolic blood pressure of 90 mmHg or greater is consistent with mild hypertension. Such patients are candidates for a trial of management without drugs that employs weight loss, dietary salt restriction, and exercise. A strong family history of hypertension and cardiovascular disease, however, may sway judgment to early pharmacologic therapy. At levels of 95 mmHg, pharmacologic therapy should be strongly considered.

There are five classes of drugs used to treat hypertension (Table 9.1), including (1) diuretics, (2) directly acting dilators of vascular smooth muscle, (3) calcium channel blockers, (4) angiotensin antagonists, and (5) drugs that decrease the activity of the sympathetic nervous system.

TABLE 9.1
Antihypertensive drugs

Class	Examples
Diuretics	
Thiazides	Chlorothiazide (Diuril), hydrochlorothiazide (Hydrodiuril)
Loop	Furosemide (Lasix), ethacrynic acid (Edecrin)
Potassium-sparing	Spironolactone (Aldactone), triamterene (Dyrenium)
Smooth muscle dilators	
Arterial vasodilators	Hydralazine (Apresoline)
Venodilator	Nitroglycerine
Arterial and venous dilator	Nitroprusside (Nipride)
Calcium channel blockers	
Arteriolar dilation	Nifedipine (Procardia)
Angiotensin antagonist	Captopril (Capotin)
Sympathetic depressants	See Table 9.2

DIURETICS

Diuretics, which promote the excretion of sodium through the kidneys, are important as a first-line treatment of essential hypertension because sodium is thought to be somehow involved in the pathogenesis of the disease. Also, as salt is excreted, it carries water with it, thereby reducing the volume of fluid in plasma and body tissues.

The three types of diuretics used in the treatment of hypertension all exert their effect by increasing the renal excretion of sodium. The most widely used, the *thiazide diuretics*, act on the tubules of the kidney (see Chapter 11) to inhibit the reabsorption of sodium from the renal tubules (especially the early portions of the distal convoluted tubule) back into plasma. The *loop diuretics* (furosemide and ethacrynic acid) act on the "loop of Henle" to block the reabsorption of sodium chloride. These diuretics have an extremely rapid onset of action and a more intense diuretic effect than the thiazides. They can be administered intravenously for short-term use or be given orally, although oral use is probably no more efficacious than the thiazides. Finally, the *potassium-sparing diuretics* (spironolactone, triamterene) act on the distal tubules of the kidney to facilitate the excretion of sodium while conserving body potassium. Although they are no more effective than the thiazides, they are used in patients who are at risk for problems associated with the potassium loss that can accompany use of the thiazide diuretics. The pharmacology of these drugs is discussed at length in Chapter 11.

DIRECTLY ACTING VASODILATORS

Drugs that dilate either arteries or veins reduce vascular tone and decrease blood pressure as a result of the decrease in either afterload (arterial dilators) or preload (venodilators). Nitroglycerin (see Chapter 8) is an example of a venodilator. Arterial vasodilators (Table 9.1) include hydralazine, minoxidil, diazoxide, and nitroprusside. The latter two are available in parenteral form only and are not used for chronic therapy.

Hydralazine (Apresoline), the most widely used of the directly acting arterial dilators, acts directly on the small branches of the arteries (the arterioles) just proximal to the capillaries. Such action decreases peripheral vascular resistance, increases cardiac output, and reduces arterial blood pressure. It gives patients with long-standing hypertension and a degree of heart failure an additional advantage by lowering the load against which the heart must pump. Heart rate is reflexly increased, which may be bothersome to patients with coronary artery disease. To prevent tachycardia, hydralazine often is administered with a beta-adrenergic blocker such as propranolol. Diuretics often are administered with hydralazine to prevent the sodium retention that may follow the vasodilatation.

Hydralazine is given orally for long-term management of chronic hypertension; parenteral administration is used for short-term management of acute hypertensive crises.

Minoxidil (Loniten) occasionally is used as an antihypertensive drug. Like hydralazine, it relaxes arterioles, thus producing a decrease in peripheral vascular resistance, an increase in cardiac output, and a fall in blood pressure. Reflex tachycardia is prominent unless the drug is given with a beta-adrenergic blocker. Minoxidil has a longer half-life than hydralazine does, which makes it somewhat more convenient to take on a long-term basis. It is used primarily in patients who fail to respond to diuretics and sympathetic blocker therapy. Side effects are frequent and tend to limit its use.

Diazoxide (Hyperstat), an intravenously administered arteriolar dilator, rapidly reduces blood pressure, improves cardiac output, and produces a reflex tachycardia. It is used primarily in hypertensive emergencies.

Nitroprusside (Nipride) is a potent, rapid, short-acting intravenous agent used by intravenous infusion for the control of hypertensive emergencies. It dilates arterioles but also exerts some nitroglycerinlike relaxant effects on veins. Continuous intravenous infusion is necessary, since its effects cease within minutes of infusion termination. The drug is metabolized to cyanide which is, in turn, metabolized to thiocyanate. Excessive levels of cyanide can develop after long-term, high-dose infusions, especially in patients whose ability to metabolize cyanide to thiocyanate is decreased.

CALCIUM CHANNEL BLOCKERS

The use of calcium channel blockers in treating arrhythmias and angina was discussed in Chapters 7 and 8, respectively. Because of their ability to dilate (or relax) the smooth muscle of arterioles, they often are used in the treatment of hypertension. *Nifedipine*

(*Procardia*), the most frequently used, reduces blood pressure and reflexly increases heart rate. It appears to be most effective when combined with a diuretic and a sympathetic blocking agent. However, it also appears to be useful in patients who cannot tolerate the side effects associated with sympathetic blockade (see pp. 88–89).

ANGIOTENSIN ANTAGONISTS

The enzyme renin is synthesized and stored in the kidneys and released in response to a decrease in blood flow to the kidneys, such as might be associated with narrowing of the renal artery by atherosclerosis. When released into blood, renin initiates the conversion (by a two-step process) of angiotensinogen to angiotensin I to angiotensin II, a very potent vasoconstrictor. Such angiotensin II-induced vasoconstriction results in marked increases in blood pressure. Surgical correction of renal artery narrowing, with restoration of normal renal blood flow, reduces the process of renin release, angiotensin II formation, vasoconstriction, and rise in blood pressure. This is one of the few surgically correctible causes of hypertension.

Captopril (Capoten) and *enalapril (Vasotec)* inhibit the enzyme (antiotensin-converting enzyme) that converts angiotensin I to angiotensin II. Bothersome side effects have limited the use of captopril to patients who fail to respond adequately to other antihypertensive drugs. The newer agent, enalapril, has a much lower incidence of side effects and may become more widely used. Enalapril is well absorbed orally and is bioactivated to enalaprilat, the pharmacologically active form of the drug. Enalaprilat itself is poorly absorbed when administered orally. Coadministration of a diuretic may increase the antihypertensive effectiveness of enalapril without a concomitant increase in side effects. Considering its proposed mechanism of action, one might expect enalapril to be effective only in patients whose hypertension was due to high renin levels; however, because it is also effective in low-renin hypertension, other actions may be involved also. One postulated mechanism is blockade of the enzyme Kininase which degrades bradykinin, a body peptide and a potent vasodilator. Thus, in addition to being therapeutically useful, drugs such as enalapril provide exciting insights into the mechanisms of hypertensive disease.

SYMPATHETIC DEPRESSANT DRUGS

Drugs that interfere with the function of the sympathetic nervous system (Table 9.2) either exert a depressant action on the heart or reduce the tone of vascular smooth muscle (see Chapter 2). These drugs can be classified as centrally acting antihypertensives, beta-adrenergic receptor antagonists, alpha-adrenergic antagonists, ganglionic blocking drugs, and adrenergic neuron blockers or depleters.

Clonidine (Catapres) and methyldopa (Aldomet) each reduce peripheral sympathetic vascular tone through a central action. Clonidine reduces the sympathetic outflow from the brain by acting on alpha$_2$ receptors in the medulla that are responsible for controlling vascular tone. The hypotensive effect of clonidine is produced by the fall in peripheral vascular resistance. Clonidine's usefulness is limited by side effects that may result from sympathetic blockade, such as excessive hypotension, drowsiness, constipation, dry mouth, and occasional sexual dysfunction. Rebound hypertension following cessation of orally administered clonidine is a major problems. Sympathetic hyperactivity develops within 8 to 14 hours after its abrupt discontinuation and patients must be carefully instructed not to miss even one dose of the drug. Withdrawal from clonidine should be done very gradually and be accompanied by increasing doses of other antihypertensives. The recent introduction of a clonidine-containing skin patch allows for prolonged transcutaneous absorption of the drug, eliminating the need for oral administration, reducing the likelihood of abrupt hypertensive crises as long as the patch is worn, and allowing for continued administration when oral preparations cannot be taken.

TABLE 9.2
Sympathetic depressant antihypertensives

Site of action	Mechanism of action	Examples
CNS-brainstem	Alpha$_2$-receptor blockade False transmitter production Transmitter depletion	Clonidine (Catapres) Methyldopa (Aldomet) Reserpine (Serpasil)
Beta-adrenergic receptors	Cardiac depression Smooth muscle relaxation	Propranolol (Inderol) Metoprolol (Lopressor) Nadolol (Corgard)
Alpha-adrenergic receptors	Receptor blockade on vascular smooth muscle	Prazosin (Minipress) Phentolamine (Regitine)
Autonomic ganglia	Ganglionic blockade	Trimethaphan (Arfonad)

Methyldopa (Aldomet) reduces sympathetic outflow from the brain, decreasing peripheral vascular resistance, blood pressure, and cardiac output. Drowsiness, mental depression, sexual dysfunction, and excessive hypotension are common side effects. The drug is administered orally for treatment of chronic hypertension and is usually given with a diuretic.

Reserpine (Serpasil), another antihypertensive drug, has fallen into disuse because of excessive drowsiness, lethargy, mental depression, and sexual dysfunction. It exerts its effect by depleting the body of catecholamine neurotransmitters, thereby reducing sympathetic activity.

The *beta-adrenergic blockers* have been discussed at several points through this book, which shows how wide and varied their use is in medicine. Because they depress myocardial contractility and relax vascular smooth muscle, they are effective in treating hypertension. Indeed, this is their most widespread use today. When combined with a diuretic, they effectively reduce blood pressure while producing fewer side effects than most other antihypertensive combinations. Since the introduction of propranolol (Inderal), the first commercially available beta blocker, numerous other beta-adrenergic blockers have become available—all of which appear to be equally effective as antihypertensive agents. These drugs are especially useful in treating angina pectoris. Since they further decrease cardiac contractility, they are less effective in patients with heart failure. Propranolol and labetolol are the only beta-adrenergic blockers available in intravenous form, which makes them useful in a wide range of clinical settings.

The great popularity of this group of antihypertensive drugs is most likely due to the relative infrequency of significant, undesirable side effects. As stated earlier, these side effects include bronchospasm, aggravation of congestive heart failure, bradycardia, sedation, and other less frequent problems. Recommendations for their clinical use will be found at the end of this chapter.

Peripheral alpha-adrenergic receptor blockers are seldom used as clinical antihypertensive agents today, having been largely replaced by the beta-adrenergic blockers. Alpha-adrenergic receptors are found in most blood vessels, especially those of the skin and internal organs. Blockade of these receptors relaxes these vessels and decreases blood pressure. One agent, prazosin (Minipress), occasionally is used as an alternative to hydralazine as a component of multiple-drug therapy in the long-term treatment of severe, chronic hypertension.

The *ganglionic blocking drugs* also are seldom used today because of their high incidence of side effects when used chronically and because there are much more effective agents available.

STEPWISE APPROACH TO THE TREATMENT OF CHRONIC HYPERTENSION

Table 9.3 lists recommendations for a progressive, stepwise, incremental approach to the treatment of hypertension. While the selection of an appropriate drug or drugs to treat hypertension depends upon numerous factors, this regime has been shown to be very effective. The therapeutic goal is to reduce diastolic blood pressure to below 90 mmHg or to the lowest level consistent with the tolerability of side effects of the drugs employed. For patients with mild hypertension, treatment usually begins with a thiazide diuretic. Side effects are few and the thiazides are well tolerated. If diuretics alone fail to control blood pressure adequately, a second drug is added. Today, the second drug will most likely be a beta-adrenergic blocking agent or a calcium channel blocker.

Hydralazine, a directly acting vasodilator, is often added as a third agent if blood pressure is not reduced adequately by the first two drugs. As discussed above, the thiazides and beta-adrenergic blockers tend to minimize many of hydralazine's side effects. This combination is particularly effective in cases of moderate to severe hypertension. If the above steps fail to control blood pressure, the patient probably should be hospitalized for an extensive evaluation and trial of even more potent sympathetic blocking drugs. Such an evaluation is often impossible to perform in an outpatient setting.

TABLE 9.3
Stepwise approach to treatment of chronic "essential" hypertension

Step 1:	Begin therapy with an oral diuretic (usually a thiazide)
Step 2:	If needed, add a sympathetic depressant drug First choice: Beta-adrenergic blocking agent Second choice: Calcium channel blocker with prominent smooth muscle relaxation Alternatives: methyldopa, clonidine, prazosin
Step 3:	If needed, add a vasodilator First choice: Hydralazine or minoxidil Alternative: Prazosin
Step 4:	If needed, consider an angiotensin antagonist (captopril) instead of steps 2 and 3
Step 5:	If needed, hospitalize for intravenous therapy with beta blocker (Propranolol) or vasodilators (diazoxide or nitroprusside)

READINGS

American Medical Association, "Antihypertensive Agents," in *AMA Drug Evaluations*, 6th ed., American Medical Association, Chicago, 1986, pp. 507–540.

"Antihypertensive Drugs," in A. Goth (ed.), *Medical Pharmacology*, 11th ed., Mosby, St. Louis, 1984, pp. 192–207.

Joint National Commission on Detection, Evaluation, and Treatment of High Blood Pressure: The 1984 Report. U.S. Department of Health and Human Services, PHS Pub. 84–1088, Bethesda, MD, 1984. [See also *Arch. Intern. Med.* **144**:1045–1057 (1984).]

Kirkendall, W. M., "Treatment of Hypertension in the Elderly," *Amer. J. Cardiology*, **57**:63C–68C (1986).

Lant, A., "Diuretics. Clinical Pharmacology and Their Therapeutic Use (part 1)," *Drugs*, **29**:57–87 (1985).

Perry, H. M., Jr., "The Evolution of Antihypertensive Therapy," *Amer. J. Cardiology*, **56**:75H–80H (1985).

Rudd, P., and T. F. Blaschke, "Antihypertensive Agents and the Drug Therapy of Hypertension," in A. G. Gilman, L. S. Goodman, T. W. Rall, and F. Murad (eds.), *The Pharmacological Basis of Therapeutics*, 7th ed., Macmillan, New York, 1985, pp. 784–805.

"Vasodilators and Calcium Channel Blockers," in R. M. Julien (ed.), *Understanding Anesthesia*, Addison-Wesley, Palo Alto, CA, 1984, pp. 140–148.

Vlasses, P. H., G. E. Larijani, D. P. Conner, and R. K. Ferguson, "Enalapril, a Nonsulfhyhryl Angiotensin-Converting Enzyme Inhibitor," *Clin. Pharmacology*, **4**:27–40 (1985).

CHAPTER 10

ANTICOAGULANTS

Blood within the arteries and the veins is held in a delicate balance between its ability to flow freely throughout all body tissues and its ability to coagulate when a blood vessel is injured or ruptures. Coagulation is the process whereby blood loses its fluid consistency and becomes a semisolid mass, or a clot. Immediately after a blood vessel is cut or ruptured, the amount of blood loss is reduced by a cascade of chemical reactions (Figure 10.1) that results in local vasoconstriction, adhesion of specialized blood elements (*platelets*) to the cut surface, formation of a platelet aggregate (or "plug"), and formation of the blood clot when fibrinogen is converted to fibrin,

FIGURE 10.1
Anticoagulation process.

(1) Inhibited by heparin; (2) inhibited by warfarin and derivatives; (3) irreversibly inhibited by aspirin, reversibly inhibited by indomethacin; (4) activated by strepokinase.

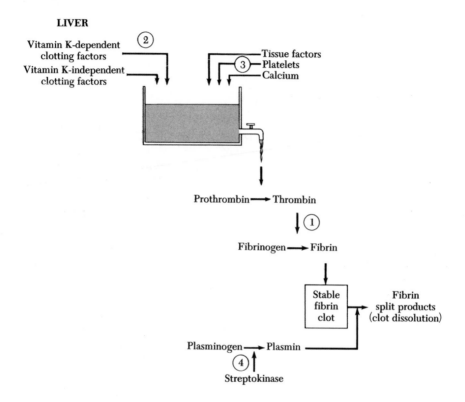

the fundamental component of the clot. The entire clotting process is well described elsewhere (see Readings) and will not be detailed here because of its complexity.

As an overview, however, note that at least six chemical reactions result in the activation of the enzyme thromboplastin which converts prothrombin to thrombin. Thrombin, in turn, catalyzes the conversion of fibrinogen to fibrin, which forms a meshwork that reinforces the already formed platelet plug and produces the final, stable clot. The chemical reactions required for the formation of thromboplastin utilize substances ("factors") that are synthesized in the liver, many of which depend on the presence of vitamin K (Chapter 18) for their formation.

Although clotting in response to tissue injury is normal and beneficial, inappropriate intravascular clotting is harmful and thought to be involved in a variety of cardiovascular disorders including deep vein thrombosis, varicose veins, and pulmonary embolism. Unwanted aggregation of platelets (platelet plugs) may be involved in strokes, heart attacks, and atherosclerosis. Finally, in patients undergoing such cardiovascular surgery as arterial bypass graphs and open heart surgery, it is essential that clot formation be prevented. Thus, anticoagulant drugs are widely used.

ANTICOAGULANT DRUGS

Drugs used clinically as anticoagulants are listed in Table 10.1. Heparin, a naturally occuring anticoagulant, usually obtained from beef lung, inhibits clotting by combining with an antithrombin to form a stable complex that increases antithrombin's ability to inactivate thrombin. Inhibition of thrombin prevents the formation of fibrin from fibrinogen and thus prevents clotting (Figure 10.1).

TABLE 10.1
Anticoagulant drugs

Drug	Action	Uses
Heparin	Inactivation of Thrombin formation	Subcutaneous to prevent venous thrombosis Intravenous to treat thromboembolism Intravenous for intraoperative anticoagulation for cardiovascular surgery
Warfarin (Coumadin), dicumerol, and others	Inhibits synthesis of vitamin K-dependent clotting factors	Long-term treatment and prevention of deep vein thrombosis and pulmonary emboli Prevention of embolus formation in patients with valvular heart disease
Aspirin and other nonsteroidal antiinflamatory drugs	Inhibition of platelet function	Long-term reduction in platelet function as prophylaxis against coronary artery occlusion and strokes in patients at risk
Streptokinase	Clot dissolution by activation of plasminogen	Dissolution of intravascular clots by local intravascular injection

Because the half-life of heparin in the body is about 1.5 hours, repeated injections or continuous intravenous infusion are necessary to maintain therapeutic blood levels and prevent thrombus formation in patients in whom the clotting process must be prevented (e.g., patients undergoing open heart surgery). In addition, "miniheparinization," about 30 to 40 percent of the full intravenous dosage, has been shown to protect against the formation of venous thrombosis in patients in risk.

When an excess dosage of heparin occurs, the result may be the major side effect of spontaneous hemorrhaging and easy bruising. Certain clotting tests, such as the partial thromboplastin time, can be used to monitor heparin therapy. Heparin is the drug of choice when an intravenous anticoagulant is necessary for early therapy, when the risk of thrombosis is high, or when it is necessary to prevent clotting in a patient for cardiovascular surgery.

Although heparin has a very short half-life, occasionally it is necessary to reduce the risk of heparin-induced hemorrhage even more rapidly. In such instances, a chemical antidote, *protamine sulfate*, is available (Table 10.2) that combines with heparin to inactivate it and block its anticoagulant effect.

Warfarin (Coumadin) and its derivatives all share an identical mechanism of action that differs from that of heparin. They block the synthesis of four essential factors in the steps of coagulation, and they do this by blocking certain chemical reactions that depend on the presence of vitamin K. These drugs have a slow onset and a fairly long duration of action and are used when anticoagulant effect is needed for a prolonged period of time. Therapy is monitored by use of the *prothrombin time*. Warfarin and its derivatives are highly bound to plasma proteins, and the levels of "free" drug in plasma vary widely depending upon the presence or absence of other drugs that are also bound by plasma proteins. Such potential for drug interactions, combined with the powerful effects of these

TABLE 10.2
Antagonists to anticoagulants

Anticoagulant	Antagonist	Comment
Heparin	Protamine	Binds with heparin to inactivate it
Warfarin-type	Vitamin K Fresh plasma	Stimulates synthesis of new clotting factors Supplies new clotting factors
Aspirin	None	Must wait for synthesis of new platelets (in emergencies one can transfuse platelets)
Streptokinase	None	None usually needed due to drug's short half-life

drugs, and their adverse effects when dosages are too high, necessitate extremely close monitoring.

Available antidotes for counteracting the actions of warfarin and its derivatives include fresh plasma, which contains the clotting factors that were inhibited by the drug, and vitamin K preparations (such as Aquamephyton), administered either intramuscularly or intravenously.

Aspirin and other nonsteroidal anti-inflammatory drugs such as indomethacin also exert antiplatelet effects. Because of this, it was thought that such drugs might be useful in the long-term prevention of clot-related cardiovascular diseases such as heart attacks and strokes. While data are still open to long-term scrutiny, aspirin is widely used and accepted for reducing of the risk of stroke in patients at risk. Whether aspirin will decrease the risk of repeat heart attacks is still not clear.

What happens to a blood clot once it is formed? Blood contains certain fibrinolytic enzymes that are capable of dissolving formed blood clots. A precursor substance, plasminogen, is activated to a substance called *plasmin* (*fibrinolysin*) which can lyse fresh clots with the production of fibrin split products (Figure 10.1). The enzyme streptokinase, a plasminogen activator, increases the availability of plasmin and thus increases clot dissolution. Streptokinase currently is approved for use in the treatment for acute pulmonary emboli, deep vein thrombosis, coronary artery occlusion, acute arterial thrombosis, and acute occlusion of vascular bypass graphs. Streptokinase is given either intravenously or intra-arterially near the site of occlusion. After initial clot lysis, clot formation should be further prevented by the use of first heparin then warfarin therapy.

READINGS

American Medical Association, "Agents Used for Anticoagulant Therapy," *AMA Drug Evaluations*, 6th ed., American Medical Association, Chicago, 1986, pp. 603–616.

Fischbach, D. P., and R. P. Fogdall, *Coagulation: The Essentials*, Williams & Wilkins, Baltimore, 1981.

Ogston, D., *The Physiology of Hemostasis*, Harvard University Press, Cambridge, MA, 1983.

O'Reilly, R. A., "Anticoagulant, Antithrombotic, and Thrombolytic Drugs," in A. G. Gilman, L. S. Goodman, T. W. Rall, and F. Murad (eds.), *The Pharmacological Basis of Therapeutics*, 7th ed., Macmillan, New York, 1985, pp. 1338–1359.

DRUG EFFECTS ON
THE KIDNEY, LUNGS, AND
GASTROINTESTINAL TRACT

CHAPTER 11

DRUGS AND THE KIDNEY

The kidneys, a pair of bean-shaped organs weighing about 150 grams (g) apiece, lie at the rear of the abdominal cavity on either side of the vertebral column (Julien, 1985, pp. 19–21). The *nephron* (Figure 11.1) is the basic unit of the kidney, and there are about 1 million nephrons in each of them. Each nephron consists of a *renal capsule* and its attached *renal tubule*.

The renal capsule is composed of two parts—a clump of capillaries, called the *glomerulus*, surrounded by an expanded, double-walled cup, call *Bowman's capsule*, which covers the capillaries of the glomerulus. The first step in urine formation, glomerular filtra-

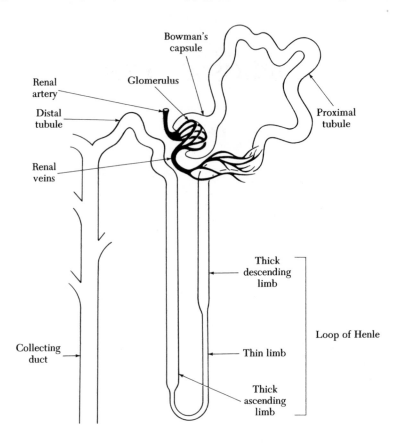

tion, occurs in the renal capsule. The hydrostatic pressure of blood in the capillaries forces a filtrate of plasma out of the capillaries into the lumen of Bowman's capsule. Such filtration is estimated to be about 120 ml per minute (about 170 l per day), enough to dehydrate a person within minutes if most of the fluid were not reabsorbed in other portions of the nephron.

Although all its sections are in continuity, the renal tubule can be functionally divided into the *proximal tubule*, the *loop of Henle*, the *distal tubule*, and the *collecting ducts*, the latter emptying into the ureters that drain into the urinary bladder. In the tubules, water and its important solutes (i.e., sodium and other electrolytes, glucose, and amino acids) are *reabsorbed* back into the capillaries (Figure 11.2) so that of the 170 l filtered each day, 168.5 are reabsorbed and only 1.5 are excreted as urine.

FIGURE 11.2
Processes involved in the formation of urine.

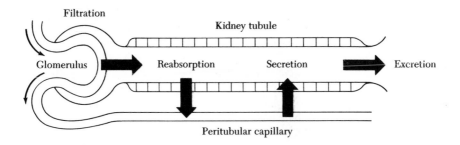

DIURETICS

Diuretics increase the renal excretion of water and sodium chloride. Their many clinical uses include removal of edema fluid, reduction in intravascular volume, and loss of sodium. In patients with cardiovascular disorders, such actions may decrease the stress on the cardiovascular system. Diuretics' uses in congestive heart failure and hypertension have been presented in Chapters 6 and 9.

Most diuretics decrease renal tubular reabsorption of sodium chloride and water either by the glomerular filtration of a substance that the renal tubules cannot reabsorb (osmotic diuretics) or, more commonly, by blocking the tubular reabsorption of sodium chloride. When sodium chloride is retained in the tubules, an osmotic equivalent of water is held also and both are then excreted. Several types of diuretics will be discussed here (Table 11.1), including thiazides, loop diuretics, potassium-sparing diuretics, osmotic diuretics, and carbonic anhydrase inhibitors. Representative structures are illustrated in Figure 11.3.

CLINICAL USES OF DIURETICS

Some of the clinical uses of diuretics include the treatment of

1. Congestive heart failure, as an adjunct to digoxin therapy
2. Hypertension, either as sole therapy or in combination with other antihypertensive drugs
3. Renal failure, to increase the excretory function of failing kidneys
4. Acute states of increased intracranial pressure and in neurosurgical procedures where osmotic diuretics reduce intracranial extracellular volume and intracranial pressure

TABLE 11.1
Site and mechanism of action of diuretics

Class of drug	Site of action in kidney	Mechanism of diuretic action
Thiazides	Proximal and distal tubules	Inhibition of sodium reabsorption
Loop diuretics	Loop of Henle (thick ascending portion)	Blockade of active sodium reabsorption
Potassium-sparing diuretics	Distal portion of distal tubule (near collecting ducts)	Inhibition of active sodium-potassium exchange (sodium reabsorption and potassium secretion)
Osmotic diuretics	Proximal tubule (major site)	Osmotic retention of sodium and water in renal tubules
Carbonic anhydrase inhibitors	Distal tubules (major site)	Inhibition of sodium bicarbonate reabsorption by block of sodium exchange for hydrogen ions

FIGURE 11.3
Structures of representative diuretic agents.

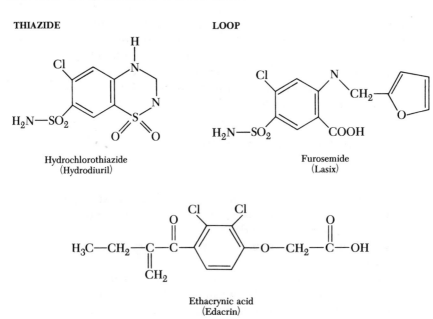

THIAZIDE

Hydrochlorothiazide
(Hydrodiuril)

LOOP

Furosemide
(Lasix)

Ethacrynic acid
(Edacrin)

FIGURE 11.3 *(continued)*

POTASSIUM-SPARING

Spironolactone
(Aldactone)

Triamterne
(Dyazide)

OSMOTIC

Mannitol

CARBONIC ANHYDRASE INHIBITOR

Acetazolanide
(Diamox)

5. Hepatic failure, to aid in the excretion of intra-abdominal fluid (ascites) that can result from such failure
6. Glaucoma, where carbonic anhydrase inhibitor diuretics reduce the formation of intraoccular fluids, which lowers intraoccular pressure

THIAZIDE DIURETICS

The thiazide diuretics are considered the most reliable, best tolerated, and most useful orally administered diuretics. Many thiazides are available (Table 11.2) and they differ primarily in potency

TABLE 11.2
Thiazide diuretics

Generic name	Trade name	Tablet sizes (mg)
Chlorothiazide	Diuril	250, 500
Hydrochlorothiazide	Hydrodiuril, Esidrex	25, 50
Bendroflumethiazide	Naturetin	2.5, 5, 10
Benzthiazide	Exna	50
Cyclothiazide	Anhydron	2
Hydroflumethiazide	Saluron	50
Methyclothiazide	Enduron, Aquatensin	2.5, 5
Polythiazide	Renese	1, 2, 4
Trichlormethiazide	Naqua, Metahydrin	2, 4
Chlorthalidone*	Hygroton	25, 50, 100
Quinethazone*	Hydromox	50
Metalazone*	Zaroxolyn	2.5, 5, 10

* A thiazide derivative, technically not a thiazide molecule.

and duration of action. These agents increase the urinary excretion of sodium chloride and water by inhibiting the reabsorption of sodium mainly in the distal tubules, possibly also with some effect on the proximal tubules. They also increase the urinary excretion of other ions, the most prominant of which is potassium. Consequently, the reduced plasma potassium level is one of the most common adverse effects of the thiazide diuretics. Dietary potassium supplementation or the concurrent administration of a potassium-sparing diuretic (see pp. 105–106) may counteract this effect. The thiazides usually are ineffective in patients with renal failure and may actually cause further deterioration of kidney function.

The thiazides are all well absorbed orally, and their onset of diuretic action usually occurs within 1 hour of administration. Although they may aggravate or precipitate acute attacks of gout because of a decreased secretion of uric acid into the renal tubules, they infrequently cause other side effects.

LOOP DIURETICS

At the present time, furosemide (Lasix) and ethacrynic acid (Edecrin) are the only loop diuretics available. Both block the active reabsorption of sodium chloride in the ascending limb of the loop of Henle, the site of greatest reabsorption of water and salt. Reabsorption at this site is much more effective than that which occurs in the distal tubules. Drugs that block sodium reabsorption in the loop have a much greater inherent activity than those that act on the tubules. Thus, the loop diuretics produce a much greater diuresis, with both the urine volume and the total sodium excreted being much greater. These potent agents usually are reserved for patients with more severe disorders that cannot be controlled by thiazides, such as renal failure, acute pulmonary edema, or hypertensive crises. Dosage forms for both oral and parenteral use are available.

Of the two loop diuretics, furosemide usually is preferred because of its lower incidence of serious side effects. Administered intravenously, furosemide has an onset of action that is almost immediate and that causes significant urine excretion. Administered orally, it has an onset of action that occurs within 1 hour and that lasts about 6 hours. Because potassium losses accompany sodium and water excretion, serum levels of potassium must be closely monitored. This very potent drug must be used with great caution in order to avoid volume depletion, hypotension, and reduced levels of sodium and potassium.

Ethacrynic acid is used less frequently because of its greater incidence of gastrointestinal disturbances and other, more serious, side effects.

POTASSIUM-SPARING DIURETICS

The diuretics discussed so far cause losses of potassium in addition to those of sodium and water. The potassium-sparing diuretics increase sodium and water excretion while conserving potassium. They do this by blocking a process in the distal renal tubule in which sodium is reabsorbed from the fluid in the lumen of the nephron in exchange for potassium. Drugs classified as potassium-sparing diuretics include the aldosterone antagonist spironolactone and two directly acting inhibitors of sodium-potassium exchange, triamterene and amiloride. Since only small amounts of sodium are normally reabsorbed in the distal portions of the distal convoluted tubules, the potassium-sparing diuretics are not as potent as either the loop or the thiazide diuretics. When combined with thiazide or loop diuretics, however, they reduce potassium losses, exert an additive diuretic effect, and are better tolerated than are potassium supplements.

Spironolactone (Aldactone), a steroid that antagonizes the effects of aldosterone, is most efficacious in patients with high aldosterone levels, such as those with hypertension caused by elevated renin levels or patients with liver failure and ascites. Serum potassium levels must be monitored carefully during spironolactone therapy. Potassium levels may rise to unacceptable levels since the secretion of potassium into the tubules is blocked. To avoid this, spironolactone usually is administered with a thiazide or loop diuretic, although serum potassium levels must still be closely monitored. Triamterene and amiloride inhibit the exchange of sodium for potassium by a direct action on the distal tubules. Such direct action makes them more reliable as diuretics than spironolactone. Both agents are well tolerated except for their propensity to retain potassium, an effect that may result in increased serum potassium levels. Concomitant administration of a thiazide tends to block this effect. Because of the offsetting effects on potassium, the combination of one of these drugs with a thiazide diuretic is widely used.

OSMOTIC DIURETICS

Mannitol is the most widely used osmotic diuretic. Its structure closely resembles that of glucose and, like glucose, it is filtered by the glomeruli of the kidney; unlike glucose, it is not reabsorbed by the tubules into plasma. Consequently, an osmotic equivalent of water passes with the mannitol through the renal tubules to increase the volume of urine excreted.

Clinical uses of mannitol include the reduction of intracranial pressure pre- and postoperatively in neurosurgical patients. It is not used for the reduction of edema associated with heart failure or ascites. When administered intravenously, mannitol has a rapid onset and a short duration of action. Its diuretic effect depends upon the amount of the drug administered.

CARBONIC ANHYDRASE INHIBITORS

Acetazolamide (Diamox) increases sodium excretion by reducing the reabsorption of sodium bicarbonate in the proximal tubules of the kidney. Thus, sodium bicarbonate is excreted along with a volume of water. Little or no chloride is excreted. Tolerance develops to the diuretic action of acetazolamide within a few days. It is the result of excess excretion of bicarbonate, which alters acid-base balance in the body and limits the drug's diuretic effects. An unusual use of acetazolamide is in acute mountain (high elevation) sickness. High altitude exposure that results in hyperventilation increases the pH of blood and makes it more alkaline. This is accompanied by the characteristic symptoms of mountain sickness including headache, malaise, nausea, and vomiting. Acetazolamide increases the excretion of bicarbonate and lowers the blood pH toward normal; symptoms often subside. Even the severe complications of high altitude sickness (primarily pulmonary edema) often can be reduced by acetazolamide. The drug therefore allows for more rapid acclimatization.

MISCELLANEOUS DRUGS USED TO TREAT UROLOGIC DISORDERS

URINARY INCONTINENCE

Urinary incontinence can result from many physiologic and psychologic factors; thus, its pharmacologic treatment is approached from several points of view.

Anticholinergic drugs block the actions of acetylcholine on the bladder and increase the bladder's capacity by reducing the stimulus to bladder contraction. As might be expected, the use of anticholinergic drugs to decrease bladder tone is accompanied by the anticholinergic side effects discussed in Chapter 3, including constipation, dry mouth, blurred vision, and tachycardia. Anticholinergic agents used to treat incontinence (Figure 11.4) include flavoxate (Urispas), oxybutynin (Ditropan), propantheline (Pro-Banthine), and the belladonna alkaloids (atropine and hyoscyamine).

Tricyclic antidepressants, especially imipramine (Tofranil), are used widely to treat nocturnal bed wetting in children. The mechanism of action is unclear, but anticholinergic side effects are prominant and may, at least partially, contribute to the effectiveness of imipramine in this disorder.

As discussed in Chapter 1, the parasympathetic and sympathetic nervous systems reciprocally innervate most body organs, including the bladder. One would think, therefore, that if inhibition of the cholinergic system were effective in treating incontinence, adrenergic stimulation should produce a similar effect. Indeed, adrenergic stimulants such as ephedrine and phenylpropanolamine (Propadrine) may have some efficacy. Adrenergic stimulants must be used with caution in hypertensive patients.

FIGURE 11.4
Structures of drugs used for urologic disorders.

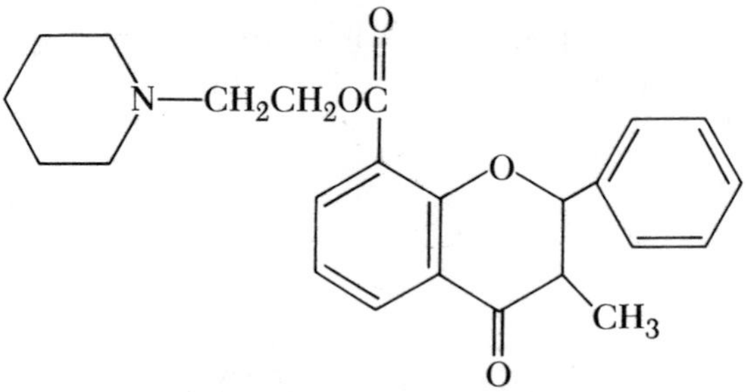

Flavoxate
(Urispas)

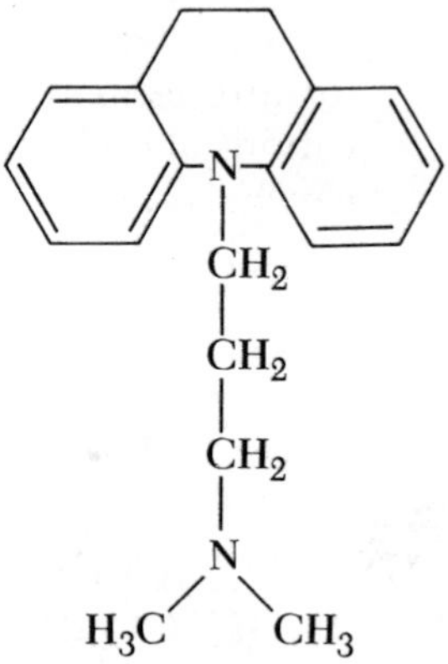

Imipramine
(Tofranil)

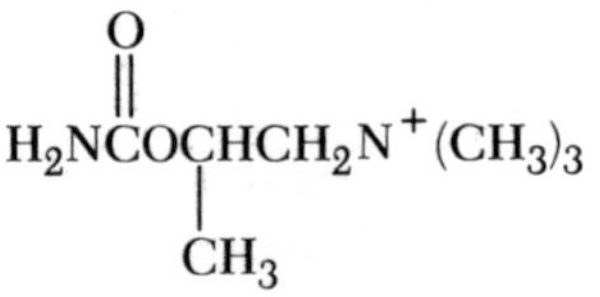

Bethanechol
(Urecholine)

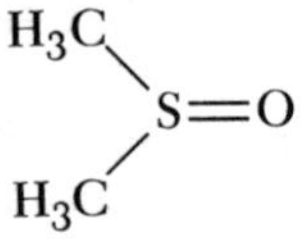

Dimethyl sulfoxide
(OMSO)

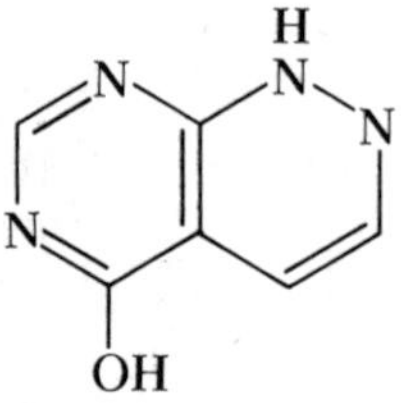

Allopurinol
(Zyloprim)

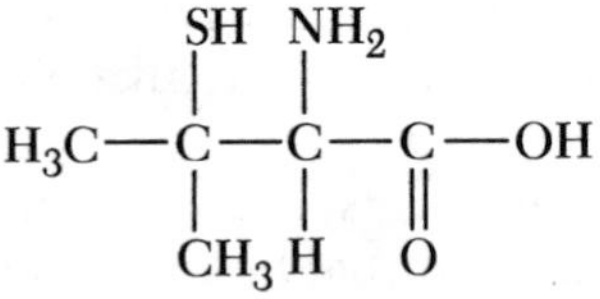

Penicillamine
(Cuprimine)

URINARY RETENTION

The reduced ability to urinate can be caused by many factors. Cholinergic stimulants and other drugs used to treat urinary retention facilitate emptying of the bladder primarily by increasing contractility. The cholinergic stimulant bethanechol (Urecholine) is widely used and clinically effective in the treatment of urinary retention.

It is most commonly used in patients with a flaccid, neurogenic bladder such as may result from spinal cord injury. It also is used occasionally in selected postoperative patients and, more recently, in patients receiving spinal injections of narcotic analgesics.

CYSTITIS

Dimethyl sulfoxide (DMSO) is an industrial solvent produced as a byproduct of the wood products industry. Although it has been tried in numerous clinical situations, it has been approved only for use in the treatment of interstitial cystitis, an inflammation of the inner lining of the bladder. Available as a 50 percent solution that is instilled directly into the bladder, it may relieve the symptoms of irritation, although such improvement is not universal. Side effects include a garlic odor on the breath, nausea, headache, and lethargy. Higher concentrations may actually cause cystitis, and an anticholinergic drug may be given simultaneously to prevent DMSO-induced bladder spasm. DMSO is held in the bladder for 15 to 30 minutes and then eliminated by voiding. Repeated treatments may be necessary.

URINARY STONES

Stones in the urinary tract are treated by dietary restriction, copious fluid intake, treatment of underlying infections, and administration of selected drugs that may reduce stone formation. The most common kidney stones are composed of uric acid. Allopurinol (Zyloprim) reduces uric acid levels by decreasing uric acid production. It does this by inhibiting one of the enzymes involved in the steps of uric acid production. Since uric acid deposits also cause symptoms of gout, allopurinol is one of the drugs of choice for treating this disorder. A different drug, penicillamine (Cuprimine), combines with the amino acid cystine to prevent the formation of cystine stones (a much rarer stone) within the urinary tract. However, this drug's side effects are numerous and serious, and it should only be used under close medical supervision.

Urinary tract infections are commonly seen disorders and are treated by antibiotics (see Chapter 19).

R E A D I N G S

American Medical Association, "Diuretics,"in *AMA Drug Evaluations*, 6th ed., American Medical Association, Chicago, 1986, pp. 541–560.

American Medical Association, "Agents Used to Treat Urologic Disorders," in *AMA Drug Evaluations*, 6th ed., American Medical Association, Chicago, 1986, pp. 567–588.

Birmingham Medical Research Expeditionary Society Mountain Sickness Study Group, "Acetazolamide in Control of Acute Mountain Sickness," *Lancet*, 1(8213):180–183 (1981).

Larson, E. B., R. C. Roach, R. B. Schoene, and T. F. Hornbein, "Acute Mountain Sickness and Acetazolamide. Clinical Efficacy and Effect on Ventilation," *J. Amer. Med. Assoc.*, 248:328–332 (1982).

Weiner, J. M., and G. H. Mudge, "Diuretics and Other Agents Employed in the Mobilization of Edema Fluid," in A. G. Gilman, L. S. Goodman, T. W. Rall, and F. Murad (eds.), *The Pharmacological Basis of Therapeutics*, 7th ed., Macmillan, New York, 1985, pp. 887–907.

CHAPTER 12

DRUGS AND THE RESPIRATORY SYSTEM

RESPIRATORY AND PULMONARY DISEASES

For purposes of discussion, respiratory and pulmonary disorders can be divided into those that affect the upper or the lower portions of the respiratory tract. The upper portion extends from the nose to the trachea, and the lower portion involves the bronchi and the alveoli of the lungs (Figure 12.1). A few remarks regarding the anatomy and physiology of these structures will help in the discussion of the pharmacologic treatment of their disorders.

FIGURE 12.1
Anatomy of the respiratory tract. (From A. C. Guyton, *Textbook of Medical Physiology*, 7th ed., Saunders, Philadelphia, 1986, p. 474.)

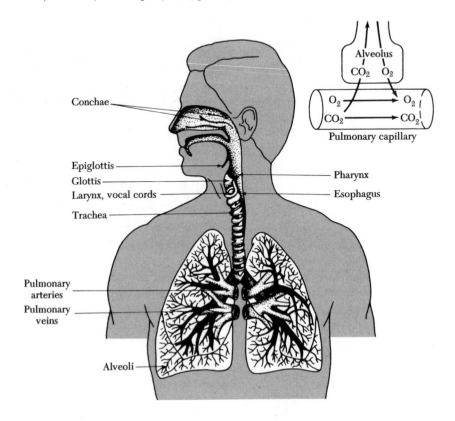

The nose functions both to warm and to humidify inspired air and to trap inhaled particulate matter. The autonomic nervous system regulates the tone of vascular smooth muscle in the nose, and this is responsible for modulating the cross-sectional area of the nasal airway. Reductions in vascular tone produce increased resistance to airflow through the nose, as is observed during exposure to cold, the common cold, inflammation or irritation of the nasal mucosa, sympathetic blocking drugs, and long-term use of nasal vasoconstrictors such as cocaine. Drugs used to treat nasal congestion are often those that *stimulate* the sympathetic nervous system or, less frequently, *block* the parasympathetic division of the ANS. Most nasal decongestants stimulate alpha-adrenergic receptors on blood vessels in the nose, constricting them and reducing both blood flow and edema in the swollen, engorged tissues. This improves the passage of air and the drainage of the sinuses. Antihistamines frequently are added to cold medications, although their role in nasal congestion is unclear. The anticholinergic side effects of antihistamines (see Chapter 4) provide a drying action which may help alleviate stuffiness. The sedation caused by the antihistamines tends to limit their use.

Acute spasm of the smooth muscle of the bronchi (bronchospasm) characterizes most lower respiratory tract disorders. Bronchospasm is considered to be a medical emergency, since air in the trachea reaches the gas-exchange membranes of the lung—thereby oxygenating blood—only after it passes through the bronchi. Narrowing or occlusion of the bronchial air passages prevents the movement of air from trachea to blood. Such bronchospastic disorders fall under the heading "asthma." The bronchial smooth muscle is dually innervated by the parasympathetic and the sympathetic nervous systems (Chapter 1) the former causing increased tone (bronchoconstriction) and the latter reduced tone (bronchodilatation). Sympathetic receptors are of the $beta_2$ type (see Chapter 2). Bronchodilators therefore either stimulate $beta_2$ receptors or closely related processes or block cholinergic receptors. Those that act by the first mechanism are therapeutically more effective.

Besides asthma, other causes of airflow obstruction in the lower respiratory tract include chronic bronchitis, which is associated with excessive mucus production and chronic cough, or emphysema, which involves irreversible damage to lung tissue. Smoking is the most usual cause of bronchitis and emphysema. Advanced states lead to reduced oxygenation of the blood (with cyanosis), respiratory difficulty, wheezing, pulmonary hypertension, and heart failure. Therapy is aimed at withdrawal from cigarettes, reducing secretions, relieving bronchospasm, and managing any infections or heart failure present. In severe cases of emphysema, supplemental oxygen may be necessary.

UPPER AIRWAY DISORDERS

Upper respiratory tract illnesses include the common cold, nasal stuffiness, membrane inflamation with cough, and bronchitis. Drugs used to treat these ailments include decongestants, cough supressants, and cold preparations.

SYMPATHETIC STIMULANTS

The majority of *nasal decongestants* are *sympathetic stimulants*, many of which are listed in Table 12.1. As a result of alpha-receptor stimulation, these drugs increase vascular tone, reduce tissue edema, increase the cross-sectional area for air passage, decrease the resistence to airflow, and improve sinus drainage. Sympathetic

TABLE 12.1
Nasal decongestants

Drug	Dosage form	Comments
Phenylephrine (Coricidin, Neosynephrine, others)	Topical sprays and solutions	Long acting, minimal CNS stimulation Strengths above 0.25% are not necessary and may produce rebound stuffiness Minimal efficiency orally
Oxymetazoline (Afrin, Duration, Neosynephrine 12-Hour)	Topical sprays and solutions	Avoid excessive use to prevent rebound stuffiness Long acting
Pseudoephedrine (Sudafed, Novafed, others)	Oral tablets	Long acting At effective doses, CNS stimulation and hypertension may occur Tolerance may develop with repeated use
Tetrahydrazoline (Tyzine)	Topical solution	Rebound stuffiness Significantly more side effects than other decongestants Avoid in children
Naphazoline (Privine)	Topical sprays and solutions	Significant rebound after continued use Cardiovascular stimulation Nasal irritation Avoid in children
Epinephrine (Adrenalin)	Topical solution	Used for nasal bleeding Significant cardiovascular effects For physician use only
Phenylpropanolamine (Propadrine, others)	Oral tablets	Mild CNS effects Tolerance can develop Widely used oral decongestant of mild efficacy
Propylhexedrine (Benzedrex)	Nasal inhaler	Minimal CNS effects Not for use by children
Xylometazoline (Neosynephrine 2, Otrivin, Sinutab Long-Lasting Nasal Spray)	Topical solution and sprays	CNS stimulation Rebound stuffiness Local irritation

stimulants are widely used for the temporary relief of nasal stuffiness and inflammation and sinus congestion associated with the common cold, hay fever, allergic rhinitis, and other acute and seasonal disorders. The primary limitations to their use are their relatively short durations of action and a rebound increase in stuffiness as their effects wear off, occurring as a result of vascular relaxation. The latter problem can be quite severe when sympathetic stimulants are used repeatedly and for long periods of time. Taken orally, a generalized sympathetic stimulation results and may include cardiac stimulation and hypertension. This response is quite unusual when these agents are applied topically as drops or as sprays.

ANTIHISTAMINES

Antihistamines occasionally are used as decongestants, probably for their drying effects, but they are included more commonly as components of mixtures that include a sympathetic stimulant. Antihistamines generally have little beneficial effect and only unwanted sedation. One should not drive or operate machinery while taking antihistamine-containing preparations, as the sedation may impair judgment and motor performance.

Occasionally, *topical steroids* are needed to decrease very severe inflammation of the nasal mucosa. These drugs may be absorbed systemically from the nasal mucosa and indirectly produce adrenocortical suppression (discussed in Chapter 14). Steroids, therefore, should be used with utmost caution under close supervision by a physician.

ANTICOUGH PREPARATIONS

Coughing serves a protective function by expelling foreign material from the respiratory tract. It is also a reflex initiated by inflammation, irritation, or thick secretions. Antitussive therapy aims to relieve unwanted coughing by depressing the cough reflex. Expectorants aim to increase mucus formation, and mucolytics to liquify thickened secretions. These drugs are available in unlimited supplies as syrups, lozenges, tablets, and so on.

Antitussives usually are classified as narcotic (codeine and related compounds) or nonnarcotic (dextromethorphan). Opiate narcotics all alleviate cough through a depressant action on the cough centers in the brainstem. Their analgesic and sedative effects also contribute to a feeling of well-being. Codeine and related narcotics obviously carry all of the dependency liabilities of narcotics in general. Dextromethorphan, while effective in alleviating cough, is not analgesic and is much less likely to cause dependency.

Glyceryl guaiacolate (Robitussin and others) is the most widely used *expectorant*. It is thought to increase secretions and thus aid both in the removal of irritants and in the soothing of inflamed membranes. Its efficacy has been questioned and challenged by many authorities.

Mucolytics, including acetylcysteine (Mucomyst) and potassium iodide, are thought to liquify tenacious secretions, thereby facilitating their expectoration. Copious amounts of water, taken orally or by mist-inhalation, would probably be at least as effective, if not more.

The number of available products marketed as *cough and cold mixtures* is enormous, but the efficacy of such products is questionable. Nevertheless, many readers may wish to refer to these in order to determine their composition and to compare them with other related products. Appendix II lists most of these products.

BRONCHOSPASM

ADRENERGIC STIMULANTS

Relief of bronchospasm is essential for the treatment of asthma. Although the ideal adrenergic stimulant would be selective for $beta_2$ receptors in the lung, most stimulate both the $beta_1$ and $beta_2$ receptors. Bronchial relaxation, therefore, generally is accompanied by cardiac stimulation and hypertension. Terbutaline, albuterol, isoetharine, bitolterol, and metaproterenol (Figure 12.2) are more selective $beta_2$ stimulants than are epinephrine, ephedrine, and isoproterenol. Given by either injection or inhalation, the latter three drugs exert a potent, rapidly acting, short-lived relaxation of bronchial smooth muscle. Ephedrine also is available in oral form for more long-lasting effects. The use of epinephrine and isoproterenol in acute attacks of severe asthma is legendary and frequently life-saving; the accompanying tachycardia is considered to be an unavoidable consequence.

The more selective $beta_2$ stimulants are available in a variety of preparations (Table 12.2) that allow for oral administration, subcutaneous injection, or oral inhalation. This allows for increased convenience, more frequent administration for prolonged efficacy, and comparably less tachycardia, hypertension, vasoconstriction, and CNS stimulation.

FIGURE 12.2

Structures of representative drugs used to treat or prevent bronchospasm.

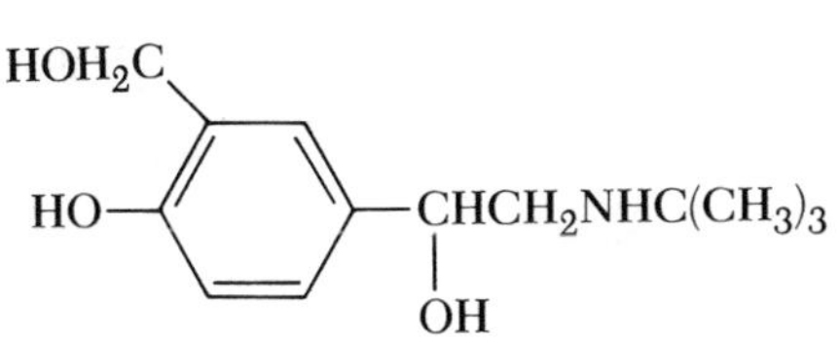

Albuterol
(Proventil, Ventolin)

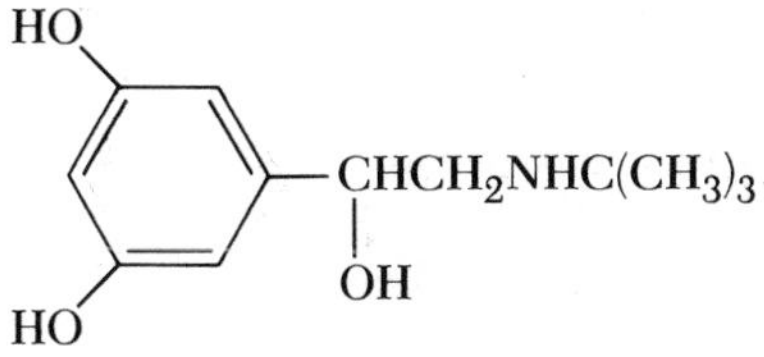

Terbutaline
(Brethine)

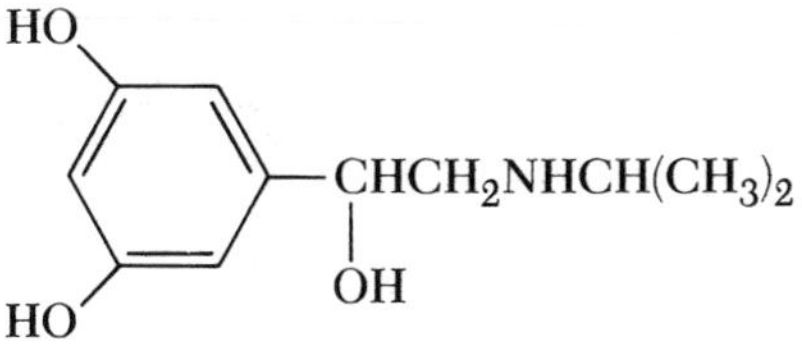

Metaproterenol
(Alupent, Metaprel)

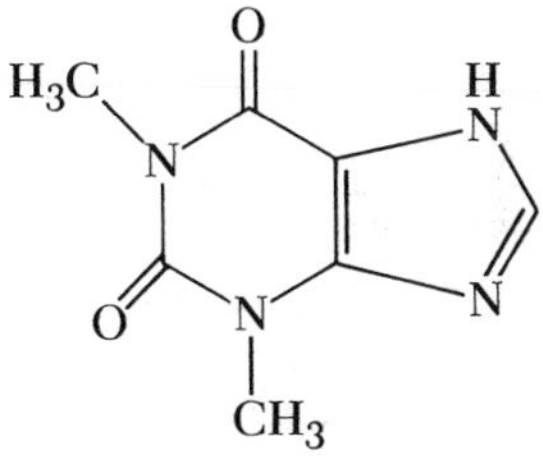

Theophylline
(Slo-phyllin, Theo-Dur, many other)

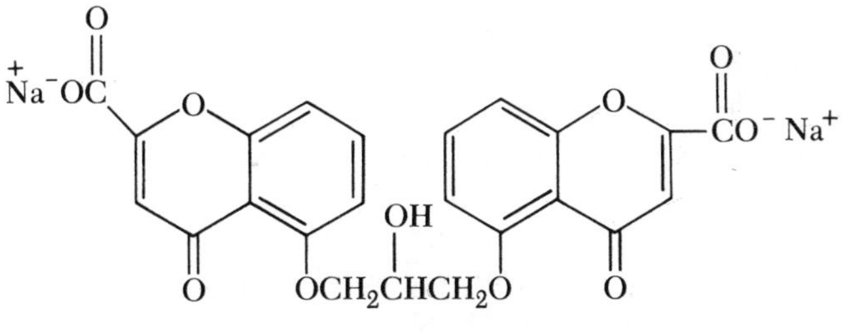

Cromolyn sodium
(Intal)

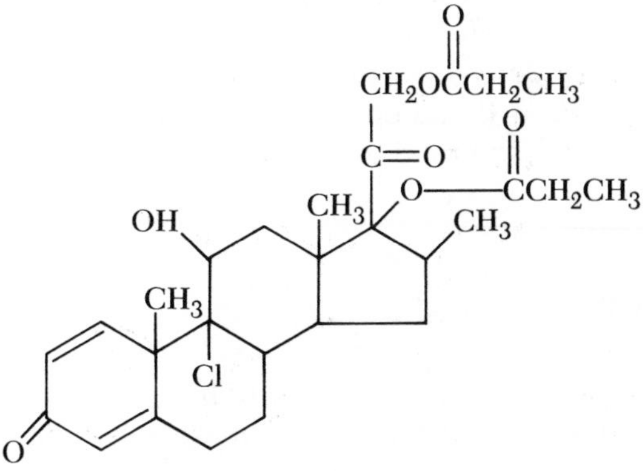

Beclomethasone dipropionate
(Beclovent, Vanceril)

TABLE 12.2
Properties of inhaled beta-adrenergic stimulants

Drug	Beta$_1$ stimulant	Beta$_2$ stimulant	Available preparations
Albuterol (Proventil, Ventolin)	+	+ + +	Metered inhaler, tablet
Terbutaline (Brethine, Bricanyl)	+	+ + +	Injection, tablet
Metaproterenol (Alupent, Metaprel)	+	+ +	Metered inhaler, tablet
Bitolterol (Tornalate)	+	+ + +	Metered inhaler
Isoproterenol (Isuprel, Medihaler-Iso, others)	+ + +	+ + +	Inhalation of solution or powder
Epinephrine (Adrenaline, Sus-phrine)	+ + +	+ + +	Subcutaneous injection
Isoetharine (Bronkometer)	+	+ +	Solution for nebulization

THEOPHYLLINE

Theophylline, the prototypical xanthine bronchodilator, produces bronchodilatation by inhibiting the enzyme phosphodiesterase and thus increasing the activity of a substance called cyclic AMP. This result is the same as would occur if the drug were to stimulate beta-adrenergic receptors directly, thereby relaxing bronchial smooth muscle. Administered either orally or intravenously, theophylline produces bronchodilatation and tachycardia, which is consistent with the beta$_1$ and beta$_2$ stimulation. A single dose of theophylline lasts several hours. Unfortunately, toxicity occurs at blood levels just above those considered to be therapeutic. The range of therapeutic concentrations of theophylline is about 10 to 20 μg/ml in plasma, and toxicity occurs when plasma levels exceed about 20 μg/ml. Sustained-release preparations of theophylline make twice or three times daily dosage possible for long-term prevention of bronchospasm. At therapeutic levels, gastrointestinal upset, tachycardia, and CNS stimulation are the most frequently occurring side effects.

CROMOLYN SODIUM

Cromolyn sodium (see Chapter 4) helps prevent bronchospasm by stabilizing the membranes of the mast cells of the lungs so that histamine release in susceptible individuals is reduced. It is quite effective, therefore, in preventing episodes of allergic asthma. Cromolyn sodium is available as a powder that is inhaled through the mouth and for use in children, as a solution that is nebulized and inhaled.

STEROIDS

Steroids are among the most potent and most effective of the antiasthma drugs. However, their systemic effects are of such importance that their use is restricted to patients who do not respond adequately to other drugs. Steroids reduce the inflammation and edema associated with bronchitis and bronchospasm, and they potentiate the effects of sympathetic stimulants and theophylline. In the presence of infection, however, they reduce the body's normal immune response.

Topical application of steroids (by inhalation) has been tried, and beclomethasone (Vanceril) is one particularly effective agent. It is well absorbed from the lungs after oral inhalation, but because it is rapidly detoxified after absorption, its systemic effects are minimized. The drug is being used increasingly as a mainstay of therapy for severe asthmatics, especially those whose asthma cannot be controlled by sympathetic stimulants or theophylline alone and in whom steroid augmentation is essential.

R E A D I N G S

American Medical Association, "Decongestant, Cough, and Cold Preparations" and "Drugs Used in Bronchial Disorders," in *AMA Drug Evaluations*, 6th ed., American Medical Association, Chicago, 1986, pp. 369–418.

Nowak, R. M., "Acute Bronchial Asthma," *Emerg. Med. Clin. North Amer.*, 1:279–293 (1983).

Owens, G. R., "New Concepts in Bronchodilator Therapy," *Amer. Fam. Phys.*, 33:218, 229 (1986).

Paterson, J. W., and R. A. Tarala, "The Treatment of Asthma. Pharmacology of Therapeutic Agents," *Med. J. Austr.*, 143:390–394 (1985).

Schleimer, R. P., "The Mechanisms of Anti-Inflamatory Steroid Action in Allergic Diseases," *Ann. Rev. Pharmacol. Toxicol.*, 25:381–412 (1985).

Shapiro, G. G., and P. Konig, "Cromolyn Sodium: A Review," *Pharmacotherapy*, 5:156–170 (1985).

Tse, C. S., and I. L. Bernstein, "Corticosteroid Aerosols in the Treatment of Asthma," 4:334–342 (1984).

CHAPTER 13

DRUGS AND THE GASTROINTESTINAL TRACT

Drugs used therapeutically for disorders of the gastrointestinal (GI) tract may be classified according to their primary use (Table 13.1). These include the prevention of gastric reflux (reflux esophagitis), treatment of peptic ulcer, relief of constipation, and relief from diarrhea.

TABLE 13.1
Drugs used to treat gastrointestinal disorders

Disorder	Drug	Mechanism of action
Reflux esophagitis	Metoclopramide (Reglan)	Increases tone of gastroesophageal sphincter Increases gastric emptying

Peptic ulcer	Antacids
	  Magnesium hydroxide (Milk of Magnesia, Aludrox, Gelusil, Mylanta)
	  Aluminum hydroxide (Amphojel, Basaljel)
	  Calcium carbonate (Titralac, Tums)
	  Dihydroxy aluminum sodium carbonate (Rolaids)
		Neutralization of gastric acids

	H$_2$ Blockers
	  Cimetidine (Tagamet)
	  Ranitadine (Zantac)
		H$_2$ blockade to reduce volume and acidity of gastric secretions

	Anticholinergics Probantheline (Pro-Banthine, many others)	Reduction in acid secretion

Constipation	Bulk Cathartics
	  Psyllium preparations (Efferylllium, Konsyl, Metamucil, Modane-bulk, Naturacil, Prompt)
	  Bran
	  Magnesium citrate
	  Magnesium hydroxide (Milk of Magnesia) } Saline cathartics
	  Fleet phospho soda
		Increased water content of stool
		Increased bulk volume of stool

	Stool softeners
	  Docusate salts (Colace, Dialose, Kasof, Modane-soft, Surfac, Doxinate)
	  Mineral oil
	  Glycerin suppositories
		Promotes water retention in stool

	Stimulant cathartics (contact cathartics)
	  Bisacodyl (Dulcolax)
	  Dehydrocholic acid (Decholin)
	  Danthron (Modane, Dorbane)
	  Senna (Senakot)
	  Phenolphthalein (Feen-a-mint, Phenolax)
	  Cascara sagrada
		Inhibition of water absorption from stool
		Stimulation of GI contraction
		Reduced transit time

(continued)

TABLE 13.1
Drugs used to treat gastrointestinal disorders *(continued)*

Disorder	Drug	Mechanism of action

Diarrhea	Narcotics
	    Tincture of opium
	    (Paregoric)
		Increased GI contractions
		    and tone
		Reduced forward movement
		    of GI contents
		Increased water absorption
		Reduced fecal volume

	Nonnarcotic GI stimulants
	    Diphenoxylate (Lomotil)
	    Loperamide (Imodium)
		Same as narcotics

	Others
	    Bulk laxatives
	    Clays (Kaolin)
		Bind water to decrease
		    watery stools

REFLUX ESOPHAGITIS

Reflux esophagitis, or *heartburn*, appears to result both from regurgitation of acid material from the stomach into the esophagus (through the gastroesophageal sphincter) and an apparent inability of the esophagus to clear the refluxed material back into the stomach. Numerous nonpharmacologic treatments help relieve heartburn, including sleeping with the head elevated, losing weight, wearing loose garments, reducing meal size, and eliminating certain foods such as coffee and alcohol.

Relief from heartburn also has been achieved by ingesting antacids (see the next section) that neutralize much of the gastric acidity, although these do little to correct the underlying disorder. Cimetidine (Tagamet) is an H_2 receptor inhibitor (see Chapter 4) that reduces the secretion of gastric acid and, for long-term therapy, is significantly more effective than either intermittent or continual ingestion of antacids. More recently, metoclopramide (Reglan) has been introduced as an even more effective drug for the treatment of reflux esophagitis. Metoclopramide (Figure 13.1) both increases the tone of the gastroesophagial sphincter and stimulates gastric emptying into the small intestine. These actions account for its clinical efficacy. Metoclopramide stimulates gastric emptying without affecting acid secretion. Its efficacy is augmented by the concurrent administration of either antacids or cimetidine. An interesting drug interaction occurs between metoclopramide and cimetidine. Because metoclopramide stimulates gastric emptying, it reduces the

FIGURE 13.1
Chemical structure of metaclopramide (Reglan).

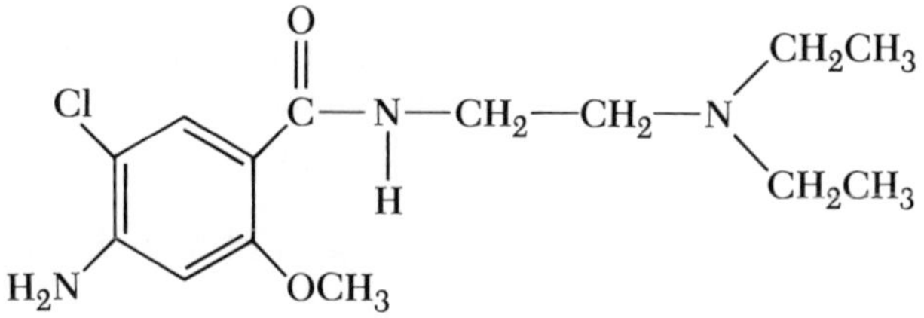

absorption of cimetidine from the stomach; therefore, either the dose of cimetidine must be increased or the drugs should be administered 1 to 2 hours apart.

PEPTIC ULCER DISEASE

Reduction of gastric acidity both promotes the healing and reduces the symptoms of ulcers occurring in either the stomach or the duodenum, the upper portion of the small intestine. Pharmacologic therapy of gastric and duodenal ulcers utilizes three classes of drugs—gastric antacids, anticholinergic drugs, and H_2 receptor antagonists.

GASTRIC ANTACIDS

Gastric antacids have been, and continue to be, the most important class of drugs in the treatment of gastric and duodenal ulcers. These aluminum, calcium, or magnesium salts (Table 13.1) react with the hydrochloric acid secreted from the stomach wall to form less acidic or even neutral products. This process of neutralization markedly reduces the pain and discomfort associated with peptic ulcer disease and facilitates healing of the ulcer.

Antacids may be subclassified as either *systemic* or *nonsystemic*, depending on the amount of drug absorbed from the GI tract. Sodium bicarbonate (baking soda) is the only systemic antacid, but it is unwise to choose to use this drug since large amounts of sodium and bicarbonate ions are absorbed into the systemic circulation. While sodium bicarbonate effectively neutralizes gastric acids, such absorption produces excess salt load, altered plasma pH, and, with prolonged use, possible acid rebound, loss of appetite, mental confusion, and muscle weakness. For these reasons, this product is not considered an appropriate drug for clinical use and it has not been included in Table 13.1

The gastric antacids of choice are the nonsystemic, or poorly absorbed, antacids. For long-term use, the various salts containing aluminum and magnesium generally are preferred over the calcium-containing antacids such as Titralic and Tums. Side effects of nonsystemic agents are relatively minor and include diarrhea with the magnesium-containing products and constipation with large doses of those containing calcium or aluminum. These products all contain widely varying amounts of sodium. In patients in whom this is of concern, such as those on a low-sodium diet for the treatment of hypertension, products with the least sodium should be chosen. Such information can be obtained from physicians or pharmacists, as product formulas are currently being revised to reflect increasing concern over this problem.

ANTICHOLINERGIC DRUGS

Anticholinergic drugs very slightly reduce the secretion of hydrochloric acid from the stomach wall. They were used for the treatment of peptic ulcers for many years, but the advent of the H_2 receptor antagonists has made them relatively obsolete. Side effects (see Chapter 3) of dry mouth, blurred vision, urinary retention, and tachycardia limit their use. Dosage usually is titrated upward until the appearance of side effects and then maintained at as high a dose as the patient can tolerate.

Representative anticholinergic drugs used to treat peptic ulcer include propantheline (Pro-Banthine), dicyclomine (Bentyl), and glycopyrrolate (Robinul). Although these drugs are now used less frequently, when administered to the point of patient tolerance and combined with regular use of antacids, they do provide relief of pain and promote healing.

H_2 RECEPTOR ANTAGONISTS

Cimetidine (Tagamet) is the prototype H_2 receptor blocker used to reduce the volume and acidity of stomach secretions. It is significantly more effective in the treatment of gastric and duodenal ulcers than either antacids or anticholinergic drugs.

A second, more potent, longer acting H_2 receptor antagonist has been introduced recently. Ranitidine's (Zantac) longer duration of action allows for twice daily dosage and, perhaps, greater patient compliance. Minimal side effects have been reported; unlike cimetidine, ranitidine does not interfere with the hepatic metabolism of other drugs, which results in a lower incidence of drug interactions. Like cimetidine, the drug is available in both oral and parenteral forms. Ranitidine appears to be a reasonable alternative to cimetidine, especially in patients resistent to the latter drug.

CATHARTICS AND LAXATIVES

Cathartics and laxatives assist the process of defecation by increasing the hydration of the intestinal contents. Although their mechanisms of action are similar, that is, both increase the water content of stool, their results differ: cathartics cause a rapid, fluid evacuation of the bowel; laxatives form soft, easily passed fecal contents.

There are relatively few indications for the use of laxatives and cathartics. Both substances are subject to wide misuse by the lay public who have many misconceptions concerning bowel function and frequency. Use of these substances is indicated for patients with such severe cardiovascular disease that excessive straining would either (1) place undue pressure on the cardiovascular system in the period preceding bowel surgery or (2) disrupt surgical sutures, and for selected patients who suffer from disorders that cause the GI tract to lose its normal contractility.

The use of cathartics and laxatives by the lay public can be curtailed by patient education, improved dietary habits, and increasing the ingestion of bulk-containing foods. The self-diagnosis of chronic constipation is *not* an indication for the continual use of these substances, as a "laxative habit" can easily result.

MECHANISM OF ACTION

Laxatives and cathartics increase the water content of feces and reduce the transit time of the intestinal contents by several mechanisms. First, the retention of water will, by hydrophylic and osmotic forces, cause an increase in the bulk of the intestinal contents and increase the rate of transit. Second, the drugs may act directly on the walls of the GI tract to block absorption of electrolytes and water and to increase the secretions into the GI tract. Third, lubricants and stool softeners act by incorporation to fecal material, retaining water and increasing the ease of evacuation.

BULK-FORMING LAXATIVES

A diet rich in fiber is an appropriate method for the prevention and treatment of most forms of constipation. The bulk-forming laxatives (psyllium preparations and bran) increase the water content and volume of the stool, which thus decreases transit time. The increased mass usually reaches the rectum within about 1 to 3 days.

Bulk-forming agents are nonabsorbed and are considered safe when adequate quantities of liquids are ingested with them. Magnesium hydroxide (Milk of Magnesia) is another bulk cathartic, but it is considerably less effective than the above agents since it retains much less water per quantity ingested.

One should note that continued constipation after adequate ingestion of bulk-forming agents (usually accompanied by a bloated and distended abdomen) may be an indication of such GI pathology as narrowing of the intestinal lumen by a tumor or other mass.

CONTACT CATHARTICS

Irritant or stimulant contact cathartics act directly on the wall of the intestine by reducing the absorption of water from the GI tract into plasma. These compounds also may stimulate the contraction of the large intestine, which reduces transit time. Contact cathartics' continuous use occasionally may produce bowel irritation or severe diarrhea that can result in dehydration and a variety of electrolyte and protein abnormalities. Such agents are best used only for short periods of time.

Agents considered to be contact cathartics include cascara, senna (more potent than cascara), danthron (Dorbane, Modane), bisacodyl (Dulcolax), and phenolphthalein. Most of these agents are available in over-the-counter preparations. Generally, they act within 6 to 12 hours and produce little or no abdominal cramping.

Dioctyl sodium sulfosuccinate (Doxinate, Colace), dioctyl calcium sulfosuccinate (Surfak), and dioctyl potassium sulfosuccinate (Dialose, Kasof) are mild contact cathartics that are widely promoted as fecal softeners. The water retention they cause effectively lessens the strain of defecation, which is useful in patients who should avoid such straining. Approximately 1 to 3 days should be allowed for full effect, since it takes that long for the softened fecal material to reach the rectum. Calcium or potassium salt products are the preferred choices for patients who must restrict their dietary intake of sodium. Diarrhea is the only adverse consequence of sulfosuccinate use, an effect that is an extention of the main use for which these drugs are intended.

MINERAL OIL

Mineral oil is a mixture of liquid hydrocarbons obtained from petroleum. The oil is indigestable and thus very poorly absorbed. It penetrates and softens the stool and may interfere with the absorption of water from the GI tract. Although it formerly was used widely, it is used less now that bulk-forming laxatives and dioctyl sulfosuccinate salts have become available.

GLYCERIN SUPPOSITORIES

Glycerin suppositories facilitate fecal evacuation within 30 to 60 minutes of insertion into the rectum. They do this by softening and lubricating hard feces located in the rectum. Glycerin suppositories are not intended for prolonged use, as more efficient stool softening can be achieved with the agents discussed above.

ANTIDIARRHEAL AGENTS

The causes of diarrhea are many and beyond the scope of the current discussion. However, severe diarrhea can cause water and electrolyte (salt) depletion and may lead to dehydration and serum electrolyte abnormalities. Hypokalemia (reduced serum potassium) can produce profound weakness and debility. Persistent diarrhea leads to severe discomfort and perianal irritation.

The management of diarrhea is based on the elimination of the cause, whenever possible, and the administration of sufficient quantities of fluids and electrolytes. The symptomatic treatment of diarrhea is justified so that temporary relief is provided until the cause is identified or the infection (usually viral) spontaneously subsides. Prolonged diarrhea may necessitate that the sufferer be hospitalized to correct the fluid and electrolyte imbalances.

Opiates have been used for the treatment of diarrhea for centuries. They increase GI contractions and increase intraintestinal tone while reducing forward propulsion of its contents—all of which serves to facilitate water absorption. Camphorated tincture of opium (Paregoric) is a traditional antidiarrheal compound. In doses most commonly used (1 teaspoonful), neither euphoria nor analgesia is produced; limited use of this preparation is not associated with an increased risk of narcotic dependennce. When used chronically, however, such a risk does exist.

Diphenoxylate (contained in Lomotil) is an opiatelike drug that is clinically useful as an antidiarrheal agent. Since the drug is virtually insoluble in water, it is poorly absorbed orally. Clinically used doses exert an antidiarrheal effect, probably by acting directly on the bowel without causing significant morphinelike systemic effects. Thus, diphenoxylate is well suited for the treatment of diarrhea when the use of more addictive opiates is undesirable.

Loperamide (Imodium), an antidiarrheal drug whose action is similar to that of diphenoxylate, prolongs transit time, increases water absorption, and reduces fecal volume. It is nearly insoluble in water and does not cross the blood-brain barrier. Because even very high doses fail to elicit the pleasurable effects typical of opiates, its overall abuse potential is lower than that of diphenoxylate. Opiates and opiatelike agents should be avoided in patients with inflammatory diseases of the bowel and in patients with liver disease.

Many other agents have been used as antidiarrheals, but none approaches the efficacy of the opiates and the opiatelike compounds. The bulk laxatives discussed above for the treatment of constipation bind water and have limited efficacy in the treatment of watery diarrhea. While the amount of stool is not decreased, frequency is reduced and stools increase in bulk. Kaolin and other clays, usually combined with pectin, are widely self-prescribed as antidiarrheals. Although they mildly reduce the fluidity of stools, total water loss is unchanged. While many of the other compounds available in over-the-counter preparations appear to do little good, they are not considered to be harmful unless they are used for prolonged periods of time or unless they delay the evaluation of potentially serious GI disorders that may underlie the cause of the diarrhea. Common sense should dictate the rational approach to self-prescribed therapy. A pharmacist can often be of valuable assistance for prescribing therapy.

For infectious diarrheas, such as those encountered as travelers' diarrhea, certain antibiotics may be used to rid the intestine of the causative organism. Because data concerning their efficacy is limited, however, and because it is possible to create antibiotic-resistent strains of bacteria, antibiotics' use should be limited to the more severe, carefully diagnosed cases. Careful evaluation by a physician is indicated before such therapy is initiated.

READINGS

American Medical Association "Gastrointestinal Agents," in *AMA Drug Evaluations*, 6th ed., American Medical Association, Chicago, 1986, pp. 937–987.

Awouters, F., C. J. E. Niemegeers, and P. A. J. Janssen, "Pharmacology of Antidiarrheal Agents," *Ann. Rev. Pharmacol. Toxicol.*, **23**:279–301 (1983).

Brunton, L. L., "Laxatives," in A. G. Gilman, L. S. Goodman, T. W. Rall, and F. Murad (eds.), *The Pharmacological Basis of Therapeutics*, 7th ed., Macmillan, New York, 1985, pp. 994–1003.

DuPont, H. L., "Nonfluid Therapy and Selected Chemoprophylaxis of Acute Diarrhea," *Amer. J. Med.*, **78**:81–90 (1985).

Hamilton, J. R., "Treatment of Acute Diarrhea," *Pediatr. Clin. North Amer.*, **32**:419–427 (1985).

Hirschowitz, B. I., "H_2 Histamine Receptors," *Ann. Rev. Pharmacol. Toxicol.*, **19**:203–244 (1979).

Kimmey, M., "Infectious Diarrhea," *Emerg. Med. Clin. North Amer.*, **3**:127–142 (1985).

Levine, J. B., "Pharmacologic Options for the Control of Peptic Ulcer Disease," *Adv. Intern. Med.*, **30**:425–447 (1984).

Paton, D. M., and D. R. Webster, "Clinical Pharmacokinetics of H_1 receptor Antagonists (the Antihistamines)," *Clin. Pharmacokinetics*, **10**:477–497 (1985).

S E C T I O N   FOUR

HORMONES AND VITAMINS

CHAPTER 14

HORMONES OF
THE ADRENAL CORTEX

The adrenal glands are small structures anatomically located on top of each of the two kidneys. They are made up of two independent parts, both of which are involved in the body's response to stress. The adrenal *medulla* secretes the catecholamines, with epinephrine being predominant (see Chapter 1). The adrenal *cortex* synthesizes and secretes two major classes of steroids—the *corticosteroids* (subdivided into *glucocorticoids* and *mineralocorticoids*) and the adrenal *androgens*.

Cortisol (Figure 14.1), the major glucocorticoid secreted by the adrenal cortex, exerts its effects primarily on carbohydrate and protein metabolism. Its potent anti-inflammatory effect has led to its wide use in the symptomatic management of rheumatoid arthritis. The rate in which aldosterone (Figure 14.1), the major mineralocorticoid secreted by the adrenal cortex, is secreted is inversely related to the dietary intake of salt. This hormone promotes salt retention. Small amounts of androgens also are released by the adrenal cortex, including dehydroepiandrosterone and small amounts of testosterone. (Most testosterone is secreted by the male testes and is responsible for masculinization of the male.)

MINERALOCORTICOIDS

Aldosterone release from the adrenal cortex is stimulated by reduction in the volume of circulating blood, by reductions in plasma sodium, and in response to the presence of angiotensin. It acts directly on the cells of the distal tubules of the kidneys to increase the reabsorption of sodium ions at the expense of potassium excretion. This produces an increase in plasma sodium, which results in water retention. The resulting increases in plasma volume, cardiac output, blood pressure, and peripheral vascular resistance are all detrimental to patients with hypertension or congestive heart failure.

FIGURE 14.1
Structures of cortisol, the principle glucocorticoid, and aldosterone, the principle mineralocorticoid, of the adrenal cortex.

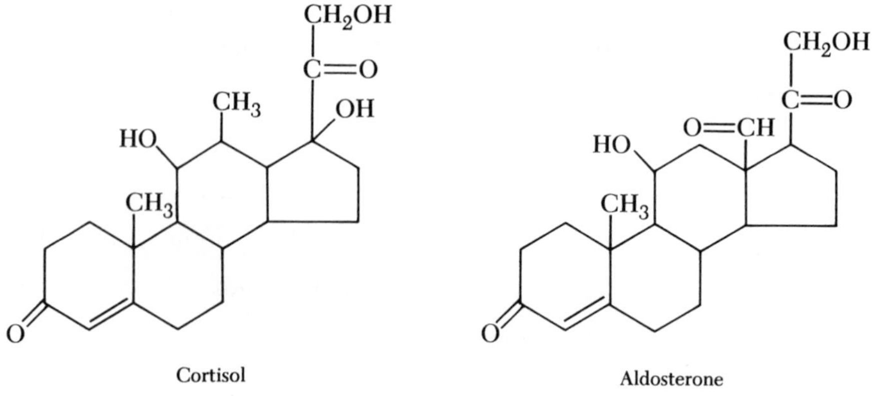

Cortisol

Aldosterone

The diuretic spironolactone (Aldactone) (see Chapter 11), antagonizes aldosterone at the level of the distal renal tubules, blocks sodium reabsorption, and promotes sodium and water excretion.

GLUCOCORTICOIDS

PITUITARY-ADRENAL RELATIONSHIPS

The synthesis and secretion of several body hormones (including the glucocorticoids) are under the influence of hormones released from the pituitary gland. The adrenal glands store very little cortisol; its synthesis and release are rapidly stimulated by corticotropin (adrenocorticotropic hormone, ACTH), a hormone released by the pituitary gland (Figure 14.2). ACTH release, in turn, is under

---

FIGURE 14.2
Hypothalamic-pituitary-adrenal involvement in cortisol secretion. Dotted line represents negative feedback inhibition of cortisol to inhibit CRF and ACTH release.

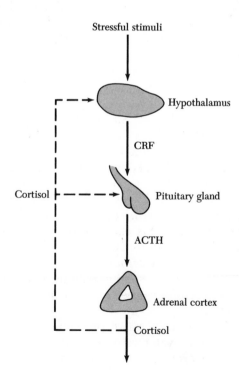

the influence of corticotropin releasing factor (CRF), a hormone synthesized in the hypothalamus and carried to the pituitary gland by a short network of veins.

The sequence of action is as follows: stressful stimuli or decreased plasma levels of cortisol are sensed by cells of the hypothalamus and result in the increased production of CRF; this induces the release of ACTH from the pituitary gland; under ACTH stimulation, cortisol is synthesized and released from the adrenal glands; increased cortisol levels (or removal of stressful stimuli) results in reductions in the release of CRF and ACTH.

Preparations of ACTH are available for intramuscular administration in slowly absorbed forms such as a gel (Cortrophin Gel; Acthar Gel) or aqueous zinc suspension (Cortrophin-Zinc). ACTH is used both to provide adrenal stimulation and to determine adrenal response to stimulation. A synthetic ACTH-like product, Cosyntropin (Cortrosyn), is available and lowers the risk of allergic reactions to the naturally occurring product.

PHYSIOLOGIC EFFECTS

Cortisol (hydrocortisone), the principal glucocorticoid of the adrenal cortex, is released in response to ACTH and shows diurnal variation, that is, secretion increases in the early morning and decreases toward late evening. About 25 mg of cortisol is secreted per day, but this rate will increase in response to stressful stimuli.

The most important metabolic effect of cortisol is to provide increased availability of energy in the form of glucose. This is a major factor in the total body response to stress. Cortisol functions to protect glucose-dependent cerebral functions by increasing the formation of glucose from body proteins, by promoting its storage in the liver as glycogen, and by decreasing its peripheral utilization.

Catabolism, the breakdown of body protein, and the inhibition of the formation of new protein are the major sources of material for glucose formation. Excesses of cortisol, as seen in Cushing's syndrome, result in wasting of skeletal muscle and loss of the protein matrix of bone. This can also occur after long-term administration of exogenous steroids. High doses of cortisol also increase body fat and alter its distribution, accounting for the "moon face" and the "buffalo hump" seen in patients with Cushing's syndrome. These metabolic effects are the opposite of the effects of insulin (see Chapter 15).

Like aldosterone, cortisol promotes the renal conservation of sodium, and thus water retention, although to much less extent than does aldosterone (Table 14.1). Cortisol promotes the renal loss

TABLE 14.1
Adrenal corticosteroids

| | Potencies as: | | Equivalent anti-inflammatory dose (mg) | Dosage forms | | |
Drug	Glucocorticoid (anti-inflammatory)	Mineralocorticoid (self-retention)		Oral	Injectable	Topical
Natural products						
Cortisol, (Hydrocortisone, Cortef, Hydrocortone)	1	1	20	x	x	x
Cortisone (Cortone)	0.8	0.8	25	x	x	
Aldosterone	0.3	1000	67	None		
Synthetic products						
Prednisone (Deltasone, Meticorten)	3	0.8	5	x		
Prednisolone (Hydeltra, Medicortelone, Delta-Cortef)	4	0.8	5	x	x	x
Triamcinolone (Kenalog, Aristocort)	5	0	4	x	x	x
Paramethasone (Haldrone)	10	0	2	x		
Dexamethasone (Decadron, Hexadrol)	25	0	0.75	x	x	x
Betamethasone (Celestone)	25	0	0.6	x	x	x
Methylprednisolone (Medrol)	4	0	5	x	x	x
Desoxycorticosterone (DOC)	0	15	0.5		x	
Fludrocortisone (Florinef)	12	100	0.02	x		
Fluprednisolone (Alphadrol)	10	0	1.5	x		

of calcium, and this, combined with the loss of bone protein, contributes to osteoporosis and fragility of bone.

ANTI-INFLAMMATORY EFFECTS

In pharmacologic doses, that is, doses greater than the equivalent amount of cortisol secreted per day, the glucocorticoids suppress the inflammatory response, alleviating the swelling, pain, and cellular destruction associated with it. The several mechanisms responsible for such action involve white blood cells, reduced capillary permeability, inhibition of prostaglandin formation, and membrane stabilization. In all instances, however, their anti-inflammatory actions relieve only the symptoms of the disease—the underlying cause eliciting the inflammatory response is unaltered.

Such reduction in inflammatory response may mask the signs and symptoms of diseases and delay proper diagnosis. It also may reduce the immune response, lowering resistance to infection and promoting its spread. Therapeutically, this reduction in immune responsiveness has led to the use of glucocorticoids to reduce the rejection of transplanted organs.

PRECAUTIONS

Adrenal corticosteroids are potent drugs with impressive effects on metabolism, inflammation, and immunity. The long-term use of pharmacologic doses produces suppression of the pituitary-adrenal axis, and such suppression may result in severe adrenal insufficiency when the drug is stopped.

The masking of infection and disease by glucocorticoids is legendary. A peptic ulcer may perforate with minimal discomfort, at least until the resulting infection becomes far advanced and possibly even fatal. Generalized infection may proceed without fever or discomfort.

Excessive use of glucocorticoids can produce Cushing's syndrome, with the accompanying osteoporosis, muscle loss, skin atrophy, peptic ulcer, altered fat distribution, hypertension, diabetic-like state, impaired immune system, and CNS symptoms of euphoria or psychotic reactions. Withdrawal is managed by prolonged, gradual reductions in glucocorticoid intake, often employing alternate-day therapy, so that adrenal insufficiency may be minimized and normal adrenal-pituitary function can resume.

USES OF GLUCOCORTICOIDS

Addison's disease results from a failure of the adrenal glands to secrete adequate amounts of cortisol (and aldosterone) to meet daily requirements. Symptoms include weakness, weight loss, loss of appetite, hypoglycemia, hypotension, and electrolyte abnormalities. Failure to secrete these hormones can be either primary, that is, the adrenals fail to secrete hormones despite adequate amounts of ACTH, or secondary to inadequate amounts of ACTH. Administration of cortisol, which is usually accompanied by another exogenous steroid with mineralocorticoid (aldosteronelike) activity, will correct the deficiency.

Rheumatoid arthritis responds dramatically to glucocorticoid therapy but use is restricted to refractory, disabling situations and even here the glucocorticoids are used only as adjuvants to nonsteroidal anti-inflammatory drugs. Although oral administration of glucocorticoids is possible, steroid dependency is often minimized by injecting the drugs directly into the most severely affected joints.

Symptoms of *allergic disorders* such as bronchial asthma are promptly relieved by glucocorticoids, although, once again, the benefits must be weighed against the adverse effects of excess dosage (with induction of a Cushingoid state) and adrenal suppression. Glucocorticoids should be used as adjuvants to other therapies in refractory patients and should be used locally whenever possible (as by inhalation in patients with bronchial asthma; see Chapter 12).

In certain *hematologic disorders*, such as autoimmune anemias and thrombocytopenia (loss of platelets), glucocorticoids may produce remission.

Certain types of *cerebral edema*, especially those resulting from brain tumors, respond dramatically to glucocorticoids. Normal cerebral function and intracranial pressure frequently are restored, at least until the tumor achieves a size in which reduction of brain edema can no longer maintain normal cerebration.

Glucocorticoids also are extremely useful in controlling the signs and symptoms of acute exacerbation of certain *collagen disorders* such as systemic lupus erythematosus (SLE), dermatologic disorders, inflammatory diseases of the bowel (such as Crohn's disease and colitis), inflammatory diseases of the liver and kidneys, and some neuromuscular disorders such as multiple sclerosis. In many of these inflammatory disorders, glucocorticoid therapy is combined with other immunosuppressive drugs (see Chapter 22).

PREPARATIONS

Synthetic glucocorticoids are all structural derivatives of cortisol (Figure 14.1). The significance of structural alterations lies in the alteration of the drugs potencies and relative ratios of glucocorticoid (anti-inflammatory) to mineralocorticoid (salt-retaining) properties (see Table 14.1).

As we stated above, local or topical application is preferred to systemic (oral or parenteral) administration whenever possible. The preparations of the various drugs available for local or systemic use are included in Table 14.1.

COMMENTS

Several points deserve summarization.

1. Glucocorticoids do not cure any disease. In Addison's disease, they provide replacement therapy. In all other states, they merely suppress the inflammatory response.
2. The inflammatory response is the body's first line of defense against infection. Glucocorticoids can cause dissemination (spread) of infections and can suppress the signs and symptoms of the spreading infection. The presence of bacterial or viral infections may be a reason for discontinuing glucocorticoid therapy. Cessation, however, can be a problem (see number 6).
3. Glucocorticoids are particularly beneficial when used short term as anti-inflammatory agents for acute flareups of inflammatory or asthmatic disease. For chronic therapy, they are much more difficult to use and possess only limited effectiveness. Usefulness is improved by topical application or by inhalation, although systemic absorption still must be considered.
4. Nonsteroidal drugs should be considered for use as first-line therapy and the glucocorticoids only for use as refractory therapy, especially when long-term use may be required.

5. Efforts always should be made to avoid and prevent production of a Cushingoidlike state.
6. Abrupt cessation of glucocorticoid therapy may result in adrenal (Addisonian) crisis and acute exacerbation of the disease for which the drug was prescribed.
7. Despite their disadvantages and limitations, glucocorticoids are of great therapeutic importance in inflammatory disorders, especially those that are chronic and disabling and those that fail to respond to other therapies.

READINGS

American Medical Association, "Agents Used to Treat Adrenal Dysfunction," in *AMA Drug Evaluations*, 6th ed., American Medical Association, Chicago, 1986, pp. 661–674.

Baxter, J. D., and G. G. Rousseau (eds.), *Glucocorticoid Hormone Action*, Springer-Verlag, New York, 1979.

Burke, C. W., "Adrenocortical Insufficiency," *Clin. Endocrinol. Metabl.*, 14:947–976 (1985).

Gold, E. M., "The Cushing's Syndromes: Changing Views of Diagnosis and Treatment," *Ann. Intern. Med.*, 90:829–844 (1979).

Haynes, R. C., and F. Murad, "Adrenocorticotropic Hormones; Adrenocortical Steroids and their Synthetic Analogues; Inhibitors of Adrenocortical Steroid Biosynthesis," in A. G. Gilman, L. S. Goodman, T. W. Rall, and F. Murad (eds.), *The Pharmacological Basis of Therapeutics*, 7th ed., Macmillan, New York, 1985, pp. 1459–1489.

Meuleman, J., and P. Katz, "The Immunologic Effects, Kinetics, and Use of Glucocorticosteroids," *Med. Clin. North Amer.*, 69:805–816 (1985).

CHAPTER 15

THE PANCREAS AND ANTIDIABETIC DRUGS

The pancreas is a glandular structure located in the mid-abdomen. It has two predominent cell types, alpha and beta, each of which synthesizes and excretes a specific hormone. Alpha cells secrete *glucagon*, a hormone with glucocorticoidlike (anti-insulin) effects in that it promotes increases in plasma glucose (primarily by the breakdown of glycogen in the liver). Beta cells elaborate the hormone *insulin*, which is a key regulator of metabolic processes, by lowering blood glucose levels and stimulating the formation of energy storage compounds (i.e., glycogen in liver and muscle cells and triglycerides in fat cells).

Insulin exerts powerful effects on glucose metabolism; its deficiency results not only in hyperglycemia (elevated blood glucose) but in many other serious derangements of fat and protein metabolism. Its release is stimulated primarily by increases in plasma glucose levels and, to a lesser extent, by certain amino acids, ketones, and hormones. Insulin acts directly on specific receptors on cell membranes to increase glucose transport across these membranes, lowering plasma levels of glucose and increasing its intracellular concentration. In liver and muscle cells, insulin also stimulates the conversion of intracellular glucose to glycogen. In fat cells it stimulates conversion of glucose to triglycerides, simultaneously inhibiting the intracellular enzymes responsible for the breakdown of these same glycogen and triglyceride compounds.

In the absence of insulin, intracellular levels of glucose fall since it cannot get from plasma across the membrane into the intracellular fluid, and energy supplies shift to the use of stored glycogen and triglycerides. Body metabolism then shifts from the utilization of sugars to the utilization of proteins and fats—the net result being the conversion of protein to glucose and fats to fatty acids and the production of ketones as byproducts.

Diabetes mellitus (sugar diabetes) is a disease caused by inadequate secretion of insulin by the beta cells of the pancreas. The most common signs of diabetes mellitus are elevations in blood glucose and a spillover of glucose into the urine. This causes increased urination, since the excreted glucose acts as an osmotic diuretic, carrying water with it. Another serious symptom includes a metabolic acidosis (*ketoacidosis*) resulting from the increased breakdown of fats (triglycerides) to acetone and acetic acid. These ketones often can be smelled on the breath, and the acidosis stimulates respiratory rate in the body's attempt to restore a normal acid-base balance. Less well understood is the essential role of insulin in preventing vascular disease. Diabetic patients have a higher incidence of cardiovascular, atherosclerotic, coronary artery, and occlusive disease of small blood vessels. Occlusive disease is evidenced by retinal damage in the eyes and the kidney damage that may accompany advanced states of diabetes.

There are two distinct types of diabetes mellitus—insulin-dependent and noninsulin-dependent diabetes. Insulin-dependent diabetes mellitus (IDDM, formerly called juvenile-onset diabetes) has an onset before adulthood and is associated with a complete lack of insulin secretion and relatively severe disease. Non-insulin-dependent diabetes mellitus (NIDDM; formerly called maturity- or adult-onset diabetes) usually develops in patients over 40 years of age and is associated with a deficiency in the ability to release endogenous stores of insulin from the pancreas, a relative insensitivity of cells to insulin, and a slower onset and a lower severity of symptoms. IDDM requires injection of exogenous insulin for control of symptoms and the maintenance of life. Dietary control combined with exercise and occasionally with oral hypoglycemic drugs (discussed later in this chapter) often are sufficient to control NIDDM, although patients sometimes may require supplemental insulin injections to control hyperglycemic episodes.

INSULIN

Insulin is a polypeptide (protein) hormone (Figure 15.1) consisting of two chains of amino acids linked by two-sulfur (disulfide) bridges. Its half-life in plasma is about 10 minutes, and its metabolization occurs in the liver and the kidneys. An appropriate *amount* and *dosage form* must be chosen for use by injection by diabetic patients. Dosage is calculated in *units* of drug. The standardization of units is based on the ability of the drug to lower blood glucose levels in laboratory animals. Most commercial insulin preparations are now packaged with 100 units of insulin per milliliter of injectable liquid. The sources of insulin are discussed below.

Variations in dosage form affect insulin's rate of absorption from subcutaneous injection sites into the systemic circulation. Some insulin preparations are listed in Table 15.1; they are divided into three groups—rapid-, intermediate-, and long-acting. The ideal insulin would be one that has a rapid onset (1 to 2 hours) and a moderately prolonged duration of action (about 24 hours). Since this ideal drug is not available, a combination of rapid- and long-acting preparations frequently suffices. A patient often injects the regular insulin and a fraction of the daily requirement of the long-acting insulin at breakfast time and the remainder of the long-acting insulin in the evening.

SOURCES OF INSULIN

Insulin preparations used to replace endogenous insulin commonly consist of the extracted and purified hormone from the pancreas glands of cattle (beef insulin) or hogs (pork insulin). Most diabetics use insulin made from a mixture of beef and pork insulin. Human insulin is now available and is used increasingly. These preparations are derived from totally synthetic processes (recombinant

FIGURE 15.1
Amino acid sequence of human insulin.

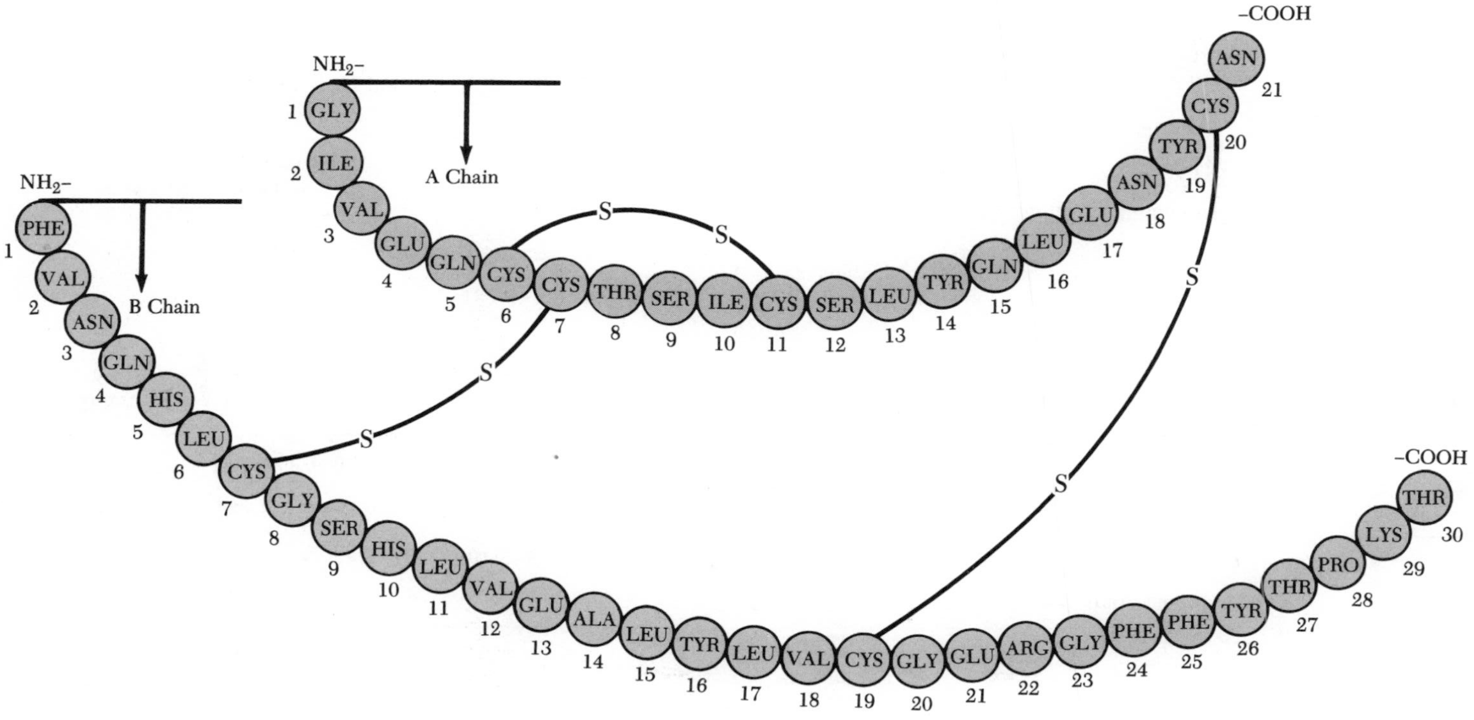

TABLE 15.1
Insulin preparations

Class	Product	Onset*	Peak*	Duration*	Source (trade name)			
					Beef	Pork	Mixed	Human
Rapid acting	Insulin injection (regular)	0.5–1	2–5	6–8	Beef Regular Iletin II	Pork Regular Iletin II	Regular Iletin I	Humulin R Novolin R
	Prompt insulin zinc suspension†	0.5–1.5	5–10	12–16	Semilente	Semitard	Semilente Iletin I	
Intermediate acting	Isophane insulin suspension (NPH)‡	1–1.5	8–12	24	Isophane Insulin NPH Beef NPH Iletin II	Pork NPH Iletin II	NPH Iletin I	Humulin N Novolin N
	Insulin zinc suspension (Lente)§	1–2.5	7–15	24	Lente Iletin II Purified Beef Insulin Zinc	Lente Iletin II	Lente Iletin I	Novolin L
Long acting	Protamine zinc insulin suspension‖	4–8	14–20	36	Protamine Zinc Insulin Beef Protamine Zinc and Iletin II	Pork Protamine Zinc and Iletin II	Protamine Zinc and Iletin I	Humulin L
	Extended insulin zinc suspension¶	4–8	10–30	>36	Ultralente Insulin		Ultralente Ilentin I	

* Hours after subcutaneous injection.

† Small particles of zinc insulin in suspension.

‡ Zinc insulin crystals modified with protamine.

§ Seventy percent extended +30 percent prompt insulin suspension.

‖ Protamine zinc and insulin in a suspension of small particles.

¶ Larger particles of zinc insulin.

DNA technology using strains of the bacterium *Escherichia coli*).*
All insulins are proteins consisting of 51 amino acids linked together (Figure 15.1). Beef and pork insulin have one or more amino
acids that differ from those of human insulin, which is a factor that
occasionally leads to allergic reactions. Pork insulin differs from
human insulin by only one amino acid and is less immunogenic
than beef preparations. Synthetic human insulin is identical to the
insulin produced by the human pancreas.

In addition to regular insulin (pork, beef, or human), other forms
of insulin have been developed to delay the onset and prolong the
duration of action. Combining insulin with a large insoluble protein
such as protamine slows absorption and prolongs the action. Preparing insulin with zinc allows for control of particle size; when
the zinc insulin crystals are modified with protamine (NPH insulin)
further prolongation of action occurs.

PRECAUTIONS

Excessive doses of insulin, especially when accompanied by reduced caloric intake, cause hypoglycemia, a fall in the level of blood
glucose. Signs of hypoglycemia include fatigue, weakness, headache, confusion, sweating, nausea, increased respiration, and hypertension. Low blood sugar may lead to convulsions, coma, and
brain damage if sugar is not given rapidly. Eating sugar or a sugar-
sweetened product usually will correct the problem and prevent
its further progression.

Other side effects include allergy, usually to the beef or pork
products; gradual development of insulin resistance, which is generally controlled by losing weight and exercising; and atrophy of
subcutaneous fat at the site of repeated injections (insulin
lipoatrophy).

ORAL HYPOGLYCEMIC AGENTS

In many patients with NIDDM, the lack of insulin lies not with its
absence from the pancreas but from its lower-than-normal rate of

* The DNA molecule is the basic building block of life; it carries genetic information
and determines the future of the cell. DNA molecules can be changed in a complex
series of scientific steps to foster the production of desired traits. In the preparation
of insulin, bacterial host cells are programmed, via the insertion of desired genes,
to produce the A and B chains that constitute the insulin molecule. Vast quantities
of these host cells may be produced by fermentation; the insulin produced is structurally identical to human insulin.

---

release from the gland and from resistance of the body tissues to the hormone. The *sulfonylureas* (Table 15.2) stimulate the secretion of insulin by the pancreas and have significant advantages over insulin for patients with NIDDM. First, they are available in tablet form, which means that patients can avoid daily injections. Second, they are more physiologic, since they release endogenous stores of the patient's own insulin. Third, allergic reactions are avoided, since insulin from animal sources is not needed.

The six oral hypoglycemic agents currently available in the United States differ primarily in duration of action (Table 15.2). It should be noted, however, that the use of these drugs may be associated with an increased incidence of cardiovascular mortality compared with patients whose NIDDM is managed by diet alone or by diet with insulin. Thus, these agents probably should be used only in NIDDM patients who cannot be controlled by diet and weight-loss programs and who are unwilling or unable to take insulin.

These drugs are not oral insulin, nor are they a substitute for insulin. They do not lower blood sugar in the patient whose pancreas does not synthesize insulin, nor are they of any value when diabetes is complicated by ketoacidosis (in such cases, taking exogenous insulin is essential). Because most patients with NIDDM are obese, diet, weight control, and exercise—all of which increase tissue sensitivity to insulin—are the primary treatments. The oral hypoglycemic agents are only adjuvants to dietary regulation.

Controversy over possible cardiovascular toxicity of these drugs has continued for the last 15 years. Experts agree that while these drugs may control hyperglycemia, they do not prevent the cardiovascular complications arising from diabetes and, in fact, may actually increase the incidence of such complications. Their benefits,

TABLE 15.2
Characteristics of oral hypoglycemic drugs

Drug	Approximate daily dosage (mg)	Half-life (h)	Duration of action (h)
Tolbutamide (Orinase)	1000	4–5	6–12
Acetohexamide (Dymelor)	500	6–15	12–24
Tolazamide (Tolinase)	250	7	10–15
Chlorpropamide (Diabenese)	250	30–36	60
Glyburide (Diabeta, Micronase)	5	10	24
Glipizide (Glucotrol)	5	2–4	10–24

therefore, must be weighed against possible adverse cardiovascular consequences. Because these agents interact with numerous other drugs that the patient may be taking (by displacing them from carrier sites on plasma proteins), and since close regulation of blood glucose is essential in diabetics, physician supervision is as important for patients taking oral hypoglycemic drugs as it is for patients maintained on insulin injections.

READINGS

American Medical Association, "Agents Used to Regulate Blood Glucose," in *AMA Drug Evaluations*, 6th ed., American Medical Association, Chicago, 1986, pp. 771–794.

Bliss, M., *The Discovery of Insulin*, University of Chicago Press, Chicago, 1983.

Boden, G., "Treatment Strategies for Patients with Noninsulin-Dependent Diabetes Mellitus," *Amer. J. Med.*, **79(2B)**:23–26 (1985).

Cryer, P. E., and J. E. Gerich, "Glucose Counterregulation, Hypoglycemia, and Intensive Insulin Therapy in Diabetes Mellitus," *New Engl. J. Med.*, **313**:232–241 (1985).

Feldman, J. M., "Glyburide: A Second Generation Sulfonylurea Hypoglycemic Agent. History, Chemistry, Metabolism, Pharmacokinetics, Clinical Use, and Adverse Effects," *Pharmacotherapy*, **5**:43–62 (1985).

Gerich, J. E., "Sulfonylureas in the Treatment of Diabetes Mellitus— 1985," *Mayo Clin. Proc.*, **60**:439–443 (1985).

Larner, J., "Insulin and Oral Hypoglycemic Drugs," in A. G. Gilman, L. S. Goodman, T. W. Rall, and F. Murad (eds.), *The Pharmacological Basis of Therapeutics*, 7th ed., Macmillan, New York, 1985, pp. 1490–1516.

CHAPTER 16

THYROID AND PARATHYROID HORMONES

THE THYROID GLAND

The thyroid gland synthesizes and releases three important hormones, two of which, *thyroxine* (T_4) and *triiodothyronine* (T_3), are involved in energy metabolism and protein formation and are essential for normal growth and development. The third, *calcitonin*, is important in the maintenance of body calcium. Calcitonin will be discussed later in this chapter, along with the parathyroid gland and its role in the regulation of body calcium. T_3 and T_4 are the topics of the present discussion.

The fundamental actions of the two major thyroid hormones, T_3 and T_4, are related to the following:

1. Production of calories (for energy utilization and expenditure)
2. Synthesis of body proteins (for normal growth and development)
3. Regulation of body temperature (by increasing cellular metabolism)

Deficiency of thyroid hormone results in reduced metabolic rate, reduced growth and development of several organ systems, and altered function of the CNS, skeletal muscles, heart, liver, kidneys, circulation, and reproductive systems. During infancy and childhood, this results in cretinism (dwarfism with mental retardation). During adulthood it results in the syndrome of myxedema (obesity, edema, puffiness of the face, muscle weakness, impaired cerebration and speech, cardiomyopathy, bradycardia, and cold intolerance). Deficiencies are treated effectively by the administration of exogenous thyroid hormone.

Excesses of thyroid hormones result either from administration of excess hormone or from excessive production of the hormones by the thyroid gland, as can occur in Grave's disease, which is a toxic goiter. Excesses often are characterized by increased heat production (with heat intolerance), tachycardia, hypermetabolism, overactivity, and protrusion of the eyeballs. Treatment is aimed at reducing thyroid hormone levels, either by decreasing the dosage of exogenous drug or by decreasing the activity of the thyroid gland.

SYNTHESIS AND REGULATION OF THYROID HORMONES

The secretion of thyroid hormones is controlled by the hypothalamus and the pituitary gland (Figure 16.1). In response to reduced levels of circulating thyroid hormone, the hypothalamus releases thyrotropin-releasing hormone (TRH) that stimulates the pituitary gland to synthesize and release thyroid-stimulating hormone (TSH). TSH, in turn, initiates the first step in T_3 and T_4 synthesis (the "trapping" of iodine by the gland) and causes the release of T_3 and T_4 from the gland. Increased levels of T_3 and T_4 in the plasma reduce TRH and TSH secretion from the hypothalamus and pituitary by a negative feedback mechanism.

FIGURE 16.1
Hypothalamic-pituary control of thyroid hormone secretion. (See text for details.)

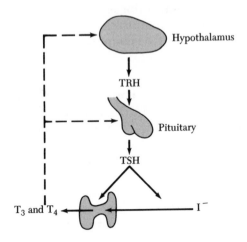

Dietary iodide from seafood or iodized salt is concentrated effectively by the thyroid gland (under TSH stimulation), which results in concentrations 30 to 200 times those found in plasma. This iodide is bound in the thyroid gland (Figure 16.2) to the amino acid tyrosine and incorporated into a large protein (thyroglobulin) as *monoiodotyrosine* (MIT) or *diiodotyrosine* (DIT). The ratio of DIT to MIT is about 10:1. Synthesis of T_3 results from the coupling of one molecule of MIT and one molecule of DIT; synthesis of T_4 results from the coupling of two DIT molecules. Normally, four times as much T_4 as T_3 is formed. The MIT and DIT are then incorporated into thyroglobulin for later release into plasma (under TSH stimulation). About 1 percent of the stored hormone is released daily into plasma. Because more T_4 than T_3 is bound by the several binding proteins, T_4 has a much longer half-life than T_3 (6 to 7 days for T_4, compared to about 2 days for T_3). The ratio of bound to free thyroxine is about 300:1.

Lack of iodine in the diet reduces the blood levels of iodide ion and the synthesis of T_3 and T_4. This results in increased release of TSH from the pituitary, which causes stimulation of the thyroid gland which is now unable to manufacture the hormone. The gland then swells and results in a *simple* or *nontoxic goiter*. Reduction in thyroid size with restoration of normal function is achieved quickly with administration of exogenous iodine or iodide salts.

FIGURE 16.2
Formation of T_3 and T_4 in the thyroid gland.

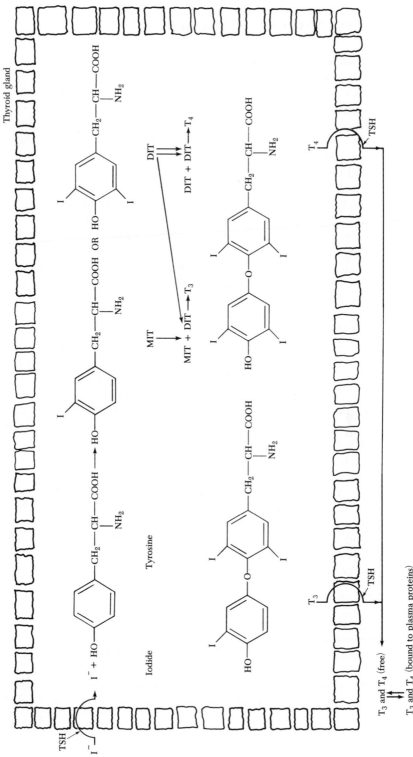

USES OF THYROID HORMONES

As stated above, iodine or iodide salts are used to treat simple goiter. About 0.1 mg per day of iodine is needed to avoid a deficiency state. Since the hypertrophied gland of a nontoxic goiter usually supplies enough hormone to meet body requirements, iodine therapy is aimed at reducing gland size so that the TSH levels may decrease and the hypertrophy may resolve. Untreated simple goiter can predispose a patient to exhaustion atropy, to hypothyroidism, and possibly to thyroid cancers.

Thyroid hormone deficiency (hypothyroidism) is treated effectively with the administration of thyroid hormones. The prototypical substance *Thyroid* is derived from the dried thyroid glands of animals. Other preparations are thyroglobulin (Proloid), synthetic salts of both T_4 (Levothyroid, Synthroid) and T_3 (Cytomel), as well as mixtures of pure T_3 and T_4 hormones (Euthyroid, Thyrolar). As might be expected, all produce similar effects but differ in source, potency, and duration of action with the T_3 product (Cytomel) having the shortest half-life.

Clinical uses of thyroid hormones include the treatment or prevention of *cretinism*, with treatment beginning in the first week of life if possible; *mild hypothyroidism*, as determined by clinical signs and laboratory confirmation; *myxedema*, to restore a euthyroid state; and *myxedema coma*, a serious sequel to, or consequence of, hypothyroidism that is characterized by hypothermia, reduced cardiac output, respiratory failure, and CNS depression. Thyroid hormones also are used to treat large nontoxic goiters and chronic thyroiditis (Hashimoto's disease, an autoimmune disease of the thyroid gland).

Thyroid hormones have no place in the treatment of obesity, despite the fact that they increase caloric utilization and have been promoted as agents that "burn fat." The dangers of excessive thyroid hormone intake (see the following section) and thyroid-pituitary–axis dysfunction far outweigh any temporary benefits obtained.

HYPERTHYROIDISM AND ANTITHYROID DRUGS

Adverse effects of excessive levels of thyroid hormone result either from the administration of excessive doses of exogenous thyroid hormone or from excessive secretion of thyroid hormone by the gland. Diseases associated with the latter include Grave's disease, toxic nodular goiter, and thyroiditis. They may represent autoimmune disorders that are characterized by excessive thyroid stimulation. Such stimulation causes thyroid hormone release that is not selflimited by the negative feedback mechanism discussed previously.

Treatment of hyperthyroidism is aimed at reducing the excessive production of thyroid hormone. Such reduction can be accomplished through the use of antithyroid drugs, radiation (radioactive iodine), or surgery (subtotal thyroidectomy). In addition, since many of the manifestations of hyperthyroidism reflect increased activity of the sympathetic nervous system, the beta-adrenergic blocking agent, propranolol (Inderal), will reduce symptoms until more definitive therapy can be instituted.

Drugs commonly used to treat hyperthyroidism include

1. Iodine, high doses of which suppress thyroid function
2. Antithyroid drugs that interfere with the synthesis of thyroid hormones
3. Radioactive iodine, which damages the thyroid gland with ionizing radiation

IODINE

Iodine is a nonmetallic basic element that is essential in body nutrition. The elementally charged component of iodine, *iodide ion*, is most commonly found as the anion in *potassium iodide*, which is added to table salt to form "iodized" salt. Iodine is the oldest remedy for both hypo- and hyperthyroidism. A daily intake of about 0.10 to 0.15 mg of the iodide ion is essential for normal thyroid hormone synthesis, which prevents the formation of simple goiter and hypothyroidism caused by its dietary lack. A large dose of iodine or the iodide ion, on the other hand, temporarily inhibits the thyroid glands and reduces the signs and symptoms of hyperthyroidism. Although the mechanism of this latter effect is unclear, it seems to involve inhibition of the synthesis and release of the thyroid hormones and suppression of iodide transport into the gland. Iodide commonly is administered as strong iodine solution (Lugol's solution) or potassium iodide solution. It is administered together with an antithyroid drug (see the following section) to prepare patients for thyroid surgery or to alleviate thyroid crisis.

ANTITHYROID DRUGS

The antithyroid drugs propylthiouracil and methimazole (Figure 16.3) inhibit the incorporation of iodide into tyrosyl residues of thyroglobulin in the thyroid hormones. (The tyrosyl residues do not become functional hormones until the iodine is incorporated.) Uses include preparation of patients for thyroid surgery, adjuvants to radioactive iodine therapy, and the chronic, nonsurgical, treatment of hyperthyroidism. Onset of action is slow because one must wait for the stored thyroid hormone to be used and the amount of hormone in the gland to be reduced. This can often take several weeks because the thyroid hormones bound to plasma proteins and stored in thyroglobulin have a long half-life. Side effects of these two drugs are relatively infrequent but potentially serious; blood dyscrasias are the most worrisome. Both drugs are well absorbed orally and undergo metabolic degradation rapidly, which necessitates frequent administration. Methimazole has a somewhat longer half-life (3 to 9 hours, compared to about 1.5 hours for propylthiouracil) and thus can be given somewhat less frequently.

RADIOACTIVE IODINE

Radioactive iodine concentrates in the thyroid gland, as does non-radioactive iodine, which causes localized destruction of thyroid tissue but not that of adjacent tissue. The most common isotope, ^{131}I, has a half-life of 8 days, and, thus, 99 percent of its radiation is expended 56 days after administration.

The drug is contraindicated in pregnancy since it crosses the placental barrier and concentrates in and destroys the thyroid gland of the fetus. Posttreatment hypothyroidism is the most common

---

FIGURE 16.3
Structural formulas of propylthiouracil and methimazole (Tapazole).

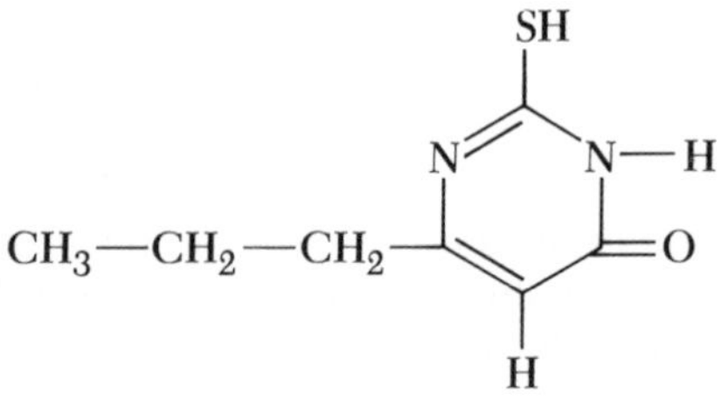

Propylthiouracil

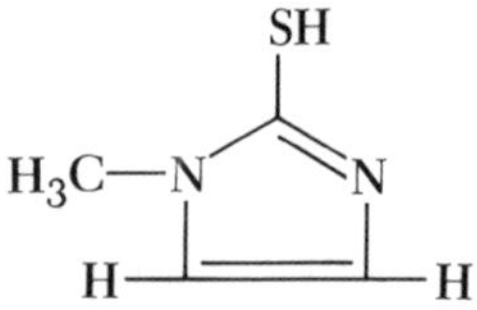

Methimazole

---

complication of radioactive iodine therapy, and it often necessitates supplemental thyroid hormone replacement. The most commonly used preparation, sodium iodide ^{131}I, is available in capsules for oral use or sterile solutions for intravenous administration. The goal of therapy is to reduce thyroid function as much as would subtotal surgical excision of the gland.

CALCITONIN, PARATHYROID HORMONE, AND CALCIUM REGULATION

The major portion of body calcium is located in bone. However, calcium plays essential roles in nerve function (excitability and transmitter release), muscle contraction, cardiac contractility and excitability, blood coagulability, and cell membrane integrity. Note that calcium's metabolic roles have priority over its structural function in bone. Thus, so that adequate plasma levels of calcium (8.6 to 10.5 mg/100 ml) are maintained, deficits will be compensated for by the resorption of calcium from bone. Other regulatory mechanisms for calcium availability include gastrointestinal absorption and renal excretion of the compound. Thus, plasma calcium is controlled by adjustments at the site of entry into the body (GI absorption) and at the site of exit (the kidneys), and by maintaining a large pool of calcium (in the bones) that is available either to make up deficits or accept excesses.

The regulation of these adjustments is complicated and involves *calcitonin* (the third hormone of the thyroid gland), *parathyroid hormone* (PTH, the hormone elaborated by the parathyroid glands, Figure 16.4), and *vitamin D*.

Calcitonin release from the thyroid gland is stimulated by a rise in the concentration of calcium in plasma. Calcitonin lowers plasma calcium by decreasing calcium resorption from bone and by increasing the renal excretion of the substance. Concomitantly, reductions in serum calcium reduce the release of calcitonin from the thyroid gland.

PTH is secreted from the parathyroid glands in response to a fall in plasma calcium. Thus it raises serum calcium by first increasing the resorption of calcium from bone, second, by increasing the renal tubular reabsorption of calcium, and, last, by increasing the GI absorption of calcium.

Vitamin D also raises serum calcium levels. Vitamin D differs from PTH, however, in that it exerts relatively greater stimulant effect on the GI absorption of calcium and on reducing its renal

FIGURE 16.4
Anatomy of the parathyroid glands in relation to the thyroid gland. The thyroid gland (right, seen from behind) wraps partway around trachea and esophagus. On the posterior surface of each lateral lobe are two parathyroid glands. (From J. V. Basmajian, 8th ed., Williams & Wilkins, Baltimore, 1982.)

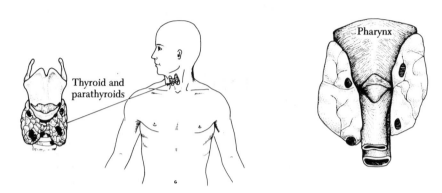

excretion. PTH stimulates the metabolism of vitamin D, which itself is inactive, into an active metabolite (1,25-dihydroxy-vitamin D). This metabolite is the major hormonal stimulant to calcium absorption from the intestine.

As discussed in Chapter 14, *glucocorticoids* also affect calcium resorption from bone and excesses can lead to osteoporosis.

Disorders of calcium metabolism involve either hypocalcemia, decreased serum levels of calcium, or hypercalcemia. Hypocalcemia, as one can predict from the discussion above, can result from inadequate calcium in the diet, vitamin D deficiency, reduced PTH secretion, and other, more subtle dysfunctions. Increased calcium intake or the addition of vitamin D, or both, often corrects the disorder, although severe disorders may require that calcium be administered intravenously. Hypercalcemia may be caused by increased secretion of PTH, vitamin D excess, certain cancers, and other diseases. Osteoporosis and renal dysfunction may manifest themselves as toxic symptoms of excessive vitamin D and the resultant hypercalcemia. The substance EDTA can chelate (bind) calcium and reduce its levels. Calcitonin (Calcimar) also may be effective.

As stated above, vitamin D excesses, in particular, lead to hypercalcemia and result in progressive weakness and fatigue, possible mental obtundation, and even coma. Renal failure, diffuse calcifications of soft tissues, and osteoporosis can follow. Thus, excesses of vitamin D can be very detrimental; levels of 2000 units or more daily should be avoided. The problems associated with overdoses of other vitamins will be discussed in further detail in Chapter 18.

OSTEOPOROSIS

Osteoporosis, a disorder involving bone calcium, is characterized by an increased rate of resorption of bone without an increase in bone formation. The resulting progressive loss of total body bone is manifested clinically by bone pain, reduced height, compression and collapse of vertebra (resulting in kyphosis), and susceptibility to fractures.

Osteoporosis is most commonly seen in postmenopausal women, especially small-statured, fair-skinned, thin women of the Caucasian and Oriental races. Factors thought to predispose people to osteoporosis include menopause with its resulting estrogen deficiency, inadequate dietary calcium and vitamin D, reduced intestinal absorption of calcium, and an increased sensitivity of bone to parathyroid hormone stimulation. The latter sensitivity (see the previous discussion) increases calcium resorption from bone, stimulates the vitamin D-induced absorption of calcium from the GI tract, and stimulates the transformation of inactive vitamin D to its active metabolite.

THERAPY

Women should assess their dietary intake of calcium in order to ascertain whether they need calcium supplements. This is especially true for postmenopausal women. A calcium intake of approximately 1 g per day is recommended, and postmenopausal women not maintained on estrogen supplementation (see the following discussion) should receive about 1.5 g of calcium daily. Small doses of vitamin D also may be indicated.

Women who have undergone hysterectomy in which the ovaries have been removed are at as great or greater a risk of osteoporosis than are those who have experienced a natural menopause. Osteoporosis seems to be more closely related to estrogen deficiency than to advancing age per se. Estrogens seem to reduce the bones' response to parathyroid hormone, which thus limits bone resorption. Women who have undergone early surgical removal of their ovaries are prime candidates for supplemental therapy with estrogen, calcium, and vitamin D. Without such replacement, bone loss can be rapid during the first few postoperative years, which increases the risk of clinically significant osteoporosis in later life. Several studies have demonstrated that the risk of fractures in postmenopausal women is markedly reduced by estrogen replacement therapy. Once significant osteoporosis has occurred, however, replacement therapy is ineffective in replacing the lost bone matrix. This therapy only inhibits bone *resorption*; it has little effect on bone *formation*.

READINGS

Ambrus, J. L., J. L. Ambrus, Jr., J. C. Robin, C. M. Ambrus, and E. A. Kahn, "Studies on the Pathophysiology and Therapy of Osteoporosis," *J. Med.*, **15**:295–309 (1984).

American Medical Association, "Agents Used to Treat Thyroid Disease" and "Agents Affecting Calcium Metabolism," in *AMA Drug Evaluations* 6th ed., American Medical Association, Chicago, 1986, pp. 795–810 and 885–902.

Boyle, I. T., "Treatments for Postmenopausal Osteoporosis," *Lancet*, **I**:1376 (1981).

Cooper, D. S., "Antithyroid Drugs," *New Engl. J. Med.*, **311**:1353–1362 (1984).

Cummings, S. R., J. L. Kelsey, M. C. Nevitt, and K. J. O'Dowd, "Epidemiology of Osteoporosis and Osteoporotic Fractures," *Epidemiol. Rev.*, **7**:178–208 (1985).

Haynes, R. C., and F. Murad, "Thyroid and Antithyroid Drugs," in A. G. Gilman, L. S. Goodman, T. W. Rall, and F. Murad (eds.), *The Pharmacological Basis of Therapeutics*, 7th ed., Macmillan, New York, 1985, pp. 1389–1411.

Haynes, R. C., and F. Murad, "Agents Affecting Calcification: Calcium, Parathyroid Hormone, Calcitonin, Vitamin D, and other Compounds," in *The Pharmacological Basis of Therapeutics*, pp. 1517–1543.

Heaney, R. P., J. C. Gallagher, C. C. Johnston, R. Neer, A. M. Parfitt, M. B. Bchir, and G. D. Whedon, "Calcium Nutrition and Bone Health in the Elderly," *Am. J. Clin. Nutr.*, **36**(5 suppl):986–1013 (1982).

Marshall, R. W., P. L. Selby, D. C. Chiluers, and A. Hodgkinson, "The Effect of Ethinyloestradiol in Calcium and Bone Metabolism in Peri- and Postmenopausal Women," *Horm. Metab. Res.*, **16**:97 (1984).

Nunez, J., and J. Pommier, "Formation of Thyroid Hormones," *Vitam. Horm.*, **39**:175–229 (1982).

Wingate, L. "The Epidemiology of Osteoporosis," *J. Med.*, **15**:245–266 (1984).

CHAPTER 17

HORMONES OF
THE PITUITARY GLAND

The pituitary gland (Figures 17.1, and 17.2) is anatomically and physiologically divided into two parts—the anterior pituitary and the posterior pituitary (the latter is also called the neurohypophysis).

The anterior lobe of the pituitary gland synthesizes and releases at least seven major hormones, all of which are under the control of *releasing factors* produced in the hypothalamus. Four of these hormones and their respective releasing factors have already been discussed: thyroid stimulating hormone (TSH) and its releasing factor (TRF) in Chapter 16; corticotropin (ACTH) and its releasing

FIGURE 17.1
Relative location of the pituitary gland in the brain.

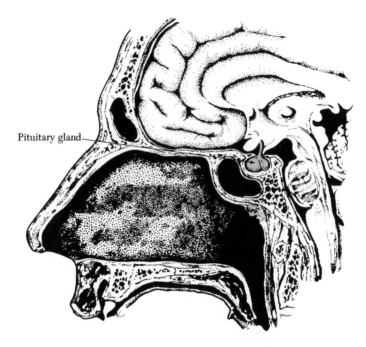

factor (CRF) in Chapter 14; and lutenizing hormone (LH) and fol-licle-stimulating hormone (FSH) and their respective releasing fac-tors (LHRF and FSHRF) in a prior volume (Julien, *A Primer of Drug Action*, 4th ed., 1985). The remaining three (growth hormone, prolactin, and beta lipotropin) will be discussed here.

The posterior lobe of the pituitary gland synthesizes and re-leases vasopressin and oxytocin, two important hormones. These compounds have important vasoactive, antidiuretic, and uterine-stimulating (oxytocic) properties. Vasopressin and oxytocin are not regulated by hypothalamic releasing factors; rather, each is syn-thesized in cells of the hypothalamus and then transported down axons to the posterior lobe of the pituitary gland where they are stored in axon terminals for later release by appropriate and some-times by inappropriate stimulation.

GROWTH HORMONE

Several hormones are essential for normal growth and develop-ment, including the thyroid hormones, insulin, and growth hor-

FIGURE 17.2
Anterior pituitary-hypothalamic hormonal relationships (a) and posterior pituitary overlying the anterior pituitary (b).

Hypothalamic releasing factors include TRH, *TSH-releasing hormone*; CRF, *ACTH-releasing factor*; LRF, *LH-releasing factor*; FRF, *FSH-releasing factor*; PIF, *prolactin-inhibiting factor*; GRF, *GH-releasing factor*; TSH, *thyroid-stimulating hormone*; ACTH, *adrenocorticotropic hormone*; LH, *luteinizing hormone*; FSH, *follicle-stimulating hormone*; PL, *prolactin*; and GH, *growth hormone*.

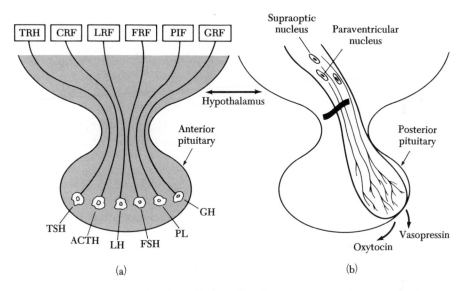

mone, estrogens (in females) and androgens (in males). Growth hormone has both growth-stimulating and protein-building properties that promote the cellular uptake of amino acids used in the manufacture of proteins.

Uncorrected deficiencies of growth hormone in childhood result in dwarfism. Formerly, growth hormone used to treat such deficiencies was obtained from extracts of human pituitary glands obtained at autopsy; 1 year of therapy required extracts from about 25 to 40 pituitaries. In October, 1985, however, the Food and Drug Administration approved and released the first genetically engineered human growth hormone (Protropin) obtained from a process of recombinant DNA manufacturing in bacteria similiar to that used to produce human insulin (see Chapter 15).

Growth hormone exerts several effects, the most important of which is related to increased cellular uptake of amino acids and to increases in plasma glucose, the latter being an anti-insulin effect. These actions appear to be mediated through poorly described compounds (somatomedins) released by the liver.

Excessive secretion of growth hormone produces such irregularities in growth as gigantism in children and acromegaly in adults. The dopaminergic stimulant bromocriptine (Parlodel) seems to inhibit growth hormone secretion from the pituitary and, in certain cases, may have some utility in the treatment of growth hormone excesses.

PROLACTIN

The primary function of prolactin, an anterior pituitary hormone, is to stimulate milk production after delivery. Other roles of prolactin in the human are only speculative at present. Suckling is the most effective stimulant to prolactin secretion.

Like other hormones of the anterior pituitary, secretion of prolactin is under hypothalamic control. This control is unique, however, in that it is primarily *inhibitory* in nature, the result of prolactin-inhibitory hormone (PIH). Dopamine (see Chapter 2) is the major CNS inhibitor of prolactin secretion and, indeed, it may be the major PIH released by the hypothalamus. Thus, as might be expected, drugs that increase dopamine activity inhibit lactation. This includes such drugs as bromocriptine, L-dopa (used in treating Parkinsonism), and clonidine (an antihypertensive drug; see Chapter 8). Conversely, drugs that inhibit dopamine activity (dopaminergic antagonists) stimulate lactation, even in nonpregnant women. This is particularly true of the phenothiazines and butyrophenones used in treating schizophrenia.

Prolactin deficiencies are rare and probably of no clinical significance except that they result in a woman's inability to secrete milk after delivery. Excesses of prolactin may result in nonstimulated milk production, menstrual irregularities, and infertility. Pituitary tumors that might cause milk secretion are treated surgically or by irradiation. Bromocriptine can be used both for a trial of pharmacologic therapy and to prevent postpartum lactation if such is desired.

BETA LIPOTROPIN

Beta lipotropin is an anterior pituitary hormone that contains the sequence for several of the "endogenous opiates," the most important of which is met-enkephalin. Whether beta lipotropin is the *source* of CNS enkephalins is unclear and probably unlikely. It may be the source of hormone fragments released from it or it may serve other, as yet unidentified, functions. Although under intensive investigation, beta lipotropin remains a "hormone in search of a function."

VASOPRESSIN

Vasopressin (antidiuretic hormone, ADH) is a polypeptide (protein) hormone containing eight amino acids. It is synthesized in cells of the hypothalamus, carried in axons to the posterior lobe of the pituitary gland, stored in nerve terminals, and released in response to alterations in plasma osmolality. Its major function is to maintain body fluid osmolality within a narrow range by regulating the excretion of water by the kidneys. Vasopressin acts directly on the renal tubules to increase the reabsorption of water by increasing the permeability of the distal tubules and collecting ducts to water. The hormone also has the ability to constrict blood vessels, which is an action that works in conjunction with the increased water reabsorption to maintain plasma volume and blood pressure.

The ingestion of large quantities of water leads to dilution of the extracellular fluid and results in decreased osmolality; this, in turn, causes inhibition of vasopressin secretion and the passive loss of water through the kidneys, which restores normal osmolality. Conversely, ingestion of hypertonic solutions leads to vasopressin release, increased water reabsorption, reduced water excretion, and reduction of the increased osmolality to normal.

Diabetes insipidus (DI) results from a deficiency of vasopressin; it is characterized by polyuria, increased water loss through the kidneys, increased concentration of plasma electrolytes, and extreme thirst (polydipsia). Patients with DI excrete large volumes of dilute urine and drink large quantities of water. DI can be caused by various means, the most common of which include head trauma, brain tumors, and other disorders that affect the posterior pituitary.

Treatment of DI requires vasopressin replacement. A variety of preparations are available, including vasopressin injection (Pitressin); vasopressin tannate injection, a suspension of vasopressin in oil, given by intramuscular injection every 2 to 3 days; and lypressin and desmopressin, both of which are administered in powder form as a nasal insufflation. Desmopressin is virtually devoid of vasoconstrictor effects, lasts 8 to 20 hours per dose, and is considered to be the drug of choice for the long-term treatment of DI.

OXYTOCIN

Oxytocin (Pitocin), like vasopressin, is a hormone of the posterior lobe of the pituitary. It is composed of a chain of eight amino acids, six of which are identical to those of vasopressin. Unlike vasopressin, oxytocin has little ADH effect and much less effect on blood vessels and blood pressure (except for a vasoconstrictive effect on umbilical vessels, which suggests that oxytocin has a role in closing umbilical vessels at birth). Oxytocin also is a potent stimulant of the pregnant uterus during and after delivery. As such it is used clinically to induce labor at term, to induce therapeutic abortion, and to prevent postpartum or postabortion hemorrhage.

Because hyperstimulation of the uterus can lead to reduced uterine blood flow, infant trauma, and even lacerations or a rupture of the cervix or uterus, close fetal and maternal monitoring is essential. The drug is contraindicated in cases of cephalopelvic disproportion, malpresentation, placenta previa, and when cesarean section is needed. It is used postpartum to induce vigorous uterine contraction and, thereby, to reduce postpartum bleeding.

Certain *ergot alkaloids* (drugs derived from the ergot fungus) are used in the postpartum period as alternatives to oxytocin. Representative agents include ergonovine (Ergotrate) and methylergonovine (Methergine). For postpartum uterine stimulation, they are administered by intramuscular injection; their effects last for several hours. Other uses of ergot alkaloids have been discussed in Chapter 4.

Other uterine stimulants used either postpartum or as abortifacients are certain of the *prostaglandins*. These can be injected either intramuscularly or into the amniotic sac, or they can be administered as vaginal suppositories. Side effects include nausea, vomiting, diarrhea, bronchospasm, and fever.

UTERINE RELAXANTS

Although not hormones, several drugs are used clinically to delay premature labor until term or at least until the fetus has matured sufficiently to survive after delivery. The adrenergic receptor stimulants of the beta$_2$ type are the most effective of currently available uterine relaxants; they have largely replaced intravenous ethanol and magnesium sulfate. The former drug both relaxes the uterus and decreases oxytocin release from the pituitary gland; the latter drug is now used primarily to prevent convulsions in patients with toxemia (eclampsia) of pregnancy.

Ritodrine (Yutopar; see Chapter 2), is another beta$_2$ stimulant that effectively relaxes the uterus when the patient is in premature labor. It usually is administered concurrently with a glucocorticoid (see Chapter 14) to aid in maturing the fetal lungs by increasing the amount of lung surfactant. When used in instances of premature labor beyond 33 weeks of gestation, ritodrine and cortisone increase the time to delivery and produce infants of greater birthweight and increased chances of survival. Ritodrine is administered either intravenously for immediate control of premature labor or orally for maintenance of uterine relaxation. Tachycardia, both in the mother and in the infant, is the most frequent side effect seen. This degree of beta$_1$ activity usually can be controlled by reducing the dosage of the drug.

READINGS

American Medical Association, "Agents Related to Anterior Pituitary and Hypothalamic Function" and "Uterine Stimulants and Relaxants," in *AMA Drug Evaluations*, 6th ed., American Medical Association, Chicago, 1986, pp. 753–769 and pp. 811–826.

Baylis, P. H., "Posterior Pituitary Function in Health and Disease," *Clin. Endocrinol. Metab.*, 12:747–770 (1983).

Caritis, S. N., "Treatment of Preterm Labor. A Review of the Therapeutic Options," *Drugs*, 26:243–261 (1983).

Vale, W., and M. Greer (eds.), "Conference on Corticotropin-Releasing Factor," *Fed. Proc.*, 44:145–263 (1985).

Franchimont, P., "Pituitary Gonadotropins," *Clin. Endocrinol. Metab.*, 6:101–116 (1977).

Frasier, S. D., "Human Pituitary Growth Hormone Therapy in Growth Hormone Deficiency," *Endocr. Rev.*, 4:155–170 (1983).

Guillemin, R., "Peptides in the Brain: The New Endocrinology of the Neuron," *Science*, 202:390–401 (1978).

Huddleston, J. F., "Preterm Labor," *Clin. Obstet. Gynecol.*, 25:123–136 (1982).

Krieger, D. T., A. S. Liotta, M. J. Brownstein, and E. A. Zimmerman, "ACTH, Beta-Lipotropin, and Related Peptides in Brain, Pituitary, and Blood," *Rec. Prog. Horm. Res.*, 36:277–344 (1980).

Murad, F., and R. C. Haynes, "Adenohypophyseal Hormones and Related Substances," in A. G. Gilman, L. S. Goodman, T. W. Rall, and F. Murad (eds.), *The Pharmacological Basis of Therapeutics*, 7th ed., Macmillan, New York, 1985, pp. 1362–1388.

Rall, T. W., and L. S. Schleifer, "Oxytocin, Prostaglandins, Ergot Alkaloids, and Other Drugs: Tocolytic Agents," in A. G. Gilman, L. S. Goodman, T. W. Rall, and F. Murad (eds.), *The Pharmacological Basis of Therapeutics*, 7th ed., Macmillan, 1985, pp. 926–945.

Richardson, D. W., and A. G. Robinson, "Desmopressin," *Ann. Intern. Med.*, **103**:228–239 (1985).

Saper, J. R., "Migraine," *J. Amer. Med. Assoc.*, **239**:2380–2383, and 2480–2484 (1978).

VITAMINS

Vitamins are organic substances that must be provided dietarily in small amounts to increase the rate of biochemical reactions within the body. They do not enter into nor are they a part of the reaction. Vitamins, therefore, are exogenous compounds required for the maintenance of life and of health.

A few other definitions are in order. A *catalyst* is a substance necessary for the performance of a chemical reaction but which remains unchanged or is regenerated while performing its task many times. An *enzyme* is a protein that acts as a catalyst for biochemical reactions in the body. In general, an enzyme can be referred to as an organic catalyst. A *coenzyme* is a partial protein that combines with another partial protein to form a complete, functional enzyme. Most vitamins act as coenzymes. In addition, they are catalysts, since they are essential for the formation, and therefore the activity, of an enzyme and do not change during the chemical reaction they foster. This explains why vitamins are required in only minuscule amounts and why their absence from the diet is associated with specific disease states.

The 13 vitamins essential for the life and health of humans can be divided into two groups: fat-soluble vitamins and water-soluble vitamins. Vitamins A, D, E, and K are fat-soluble; vitamin C and the eight B vitamins are water-soluble. The importance of fat solubility versus water solubility lies in the ability of the body either to store or excrete vitamin excesses. The fat-soluble vitamins are stored in great quantity because they are soluble in such body tissues as fat, cell membranes, liver, etc. The water-soluble vitamins are stored in only minuscule amounts, and their excesses are excreted in the urine, usually without adverse effects. Because they cannot be stored, they need to be consumed more frequently so that saturation of tissues is maintained.

Since all vitamins are obtained by the ingestion of foods, and since all vitamins are essential for health, lack of intake of any vitamin will result in a specific deficiency disorder that is reversible when the vitamin is resupplied. The deficiency state associated with each vitamin is discussed next.

VITAMIN REQUIREMENTS

In the United States, the Food and Nutrition Board of the National Academy of Sciences and the Department of Health and Human Services of the Food and Drug Administration publish recommended daily amounts of nutrients that promote good health. The recommended daily levels of vitamins are shown in Table 18.1. These levels are set high deliberately to cover the needs of virtually all healthy individuals. If the upper limits of the recommendations are maintained as a daily intake, vitamin deficiencies will be unlikely to occur. Since these are set high deliberately, intakes slightly below these levels also are unlikely to result in major deficiencies. These recommendations are intended to serve as standards for the intelligent intake of vitamins.

Many people, for one reason or another, ingest quantities of vitamins considerably in excess of these recommendations. Such

TABLE 18.1
Recommended daily intake of vitamins

Vitamins, minerals, and protein	Infants	Adults and children (>4 yr)	Children (<4 yr)	Pregnant or lactating women
Vitamin A (IU)	1500	5000	2500	8000
Vitamin D (IU)	400	400*	400	400
Vitamin E (IU)	5.0	30	10	30
Vitamin C (mg)	35	60	40	60
Folic acid (mg)	0.1	0.4	0.2	0.8
Thiamine (mg)	0.5	1.5	0.7	1.7
Riboflavin (mg)	0.6	1.7	0.8	2.0
Niacin (mg)	8.0	20	9.0	20
Vitamin B_6 (mg)	0.4	2.0	0.7	2.5
Vitamin B_{12} (μg)	2.0	6.0	3.0	8.0
Biotin (mg)	0.5	0.3	0.15	0.3
Pantothenic acid (mg)	3.0	10	5.0	10
Calcium (g)	0.6	1.0	0.8	1.3
Phosphorus (g)	0.5	1.0	0.8	1.3
Iodine (μg)	45	150	70	150
Iron (mg)	15	18	10	18
Magnesium (mg)	70	400	200	450
Copper (mg)	0.6	2.0	1.0	2.0
Zinc (mg)	5.0	15	8.0	15
Protein (g)	18†	45†	20†	

* Presence optional for adults and children 4 or more years of age in vitamin and mineral supplements.
† If protein efficiency ratio of protein is equal to or better than that of casein, U.S. RDA is 45 g for adults, 18 g for infants, and 20 g for children under 4.
SOURCE: U.S. Department of Health and Human Services, Food and Drug Administration Office of Public Affairs, Rockville, MD, revised March 1981.

nutritional supplementation in the vast majority of individuals is unnecessary, and, in a few instances, it can result in harm. For discussion of the hazards associated with excess intake of vitamins, the review by Miller and Hayes (1982) and the text by Marshall (1985) are recommended.

FAT-SOLUBLE VITAMINS

VITAMIN A

Vitamin A has a number of important functions in the body. It is essential for vision, especially in connection with adaptation to dark, and for the structural integrity of the eye. Vitamin A is necessary for the health and development of the skin as well as other cellular linings of the body. It is also essential for bone growth, sexual reproduction, and fetal development.

Sources
The average adult receives half of his or her daily intake of vitamin A as preformed vitamin (*retinol*) and the remainder as precursors to vitamin A formation (*carotenoids*). Retinol is found in liver, butter, cheese, whole milk, egg yolk, and fish. Carotenoids are present in various yellow or green fruits and in vegetables. Fish liver oils contain extremely high levels of vitamin A, and excessive ingestion of such oils can lead to toxicity.

Deficiency
Deficiencies of vitamin A can produce night blindness; thick, rough, dry, ulcerated skin; increased susceptibility to respiratory infections; dryness and thickening of the conjunctiva; and blindness.

Requirement
The recommended daily amount of vitamin A for adults is 5000 international units (IU), decreasing to 1500 IU in infants and increasing to 8000 IU in pregnant or lactating women (Table 18.1). These levels will keep individuals free of all deficiency symptoms. Given a 2500 IU daily requirement of vitamin A and a body storage of 500,000 U, an adult would have to cease the total daily intake of vitamin A for 200 days to deplete these reserves. Intakes in excess of these recommendations can lead to saturation of storage sites and eventually to accumulation to toxic levels (see the next section). Vitamin A intake over approximately 10,000 IU per day should be avoided.

Toxicities
When intake of vitamin A greatly exceeds daily requirements, a syndrome known as *hypervitaminosis A* occurs. Several hundred cases have been reported, usually in children who have received excessive amounts from well-meaning adults who wish to have "healthy" children. Signs and symptoms of chronic hypervitaminosis A include dry, itchy, and scaling skin; cracking lips; appetite and energy loss; fatigue; and irritability. The liver and spleen can become enlarged, and the liver may become cirrhotic. Intracranial pressure may increase, and neurologic symptoms may mimic those of a brain tumor. Elimination of all sources of vitamin leads to a marked reduction in symptomatology, although the skin alterations may persist for several months.

Medical Uses

Because adequate amounts of vitamin A are normally found in a well-balanced diet, supplementation usually is unnecessary. The vitamin is prescribed for patients with diagnosed vitamin A deficiency diseases, however, although such deficiencies can usually be compensated for by simply altering one's diet. During early infancy or during pregnancy and lactation, however, supplementation may be prescribed to insure that the amounts of the vitamin listed in Table 18.1 are taken in. Vitamin A also has been used to treat certain skin diseases such as acne and psoriasis, although its use should be recommended by a dermatologist.

VITAMIN D

The role of vitamin D in promoting the absorption of calcium from the intestine was discussed in Chapter 16. It should be added that vitamin D also regulates the metabolism of both calcium and phosphorus. Dietary vitamin D, or that which is synthesized by the body (in the skin), must be metabolically activated to be an active vitamin. The active form of vitamin D, *calcitriol*, is a compound formed from cholecalciferol, which is formed by the action of sunlight on a cholesterol derivative in the skin. Ideally, enough vitamin D should be manufactured by the skin to meet body requirements, but dietary ingestion of small amounts of vitamin D (about 400 IU per day) is thought to be necessary. Infants, children, and pregnant or lactating women may require up to twice this amount.

Sources

The major sources of natural vitamin D are the livers or liver oils of fish. Other sources include tuna, salmon, herring, egg yolk, and dairy products. Today, the fortification of milk with vitamin D provides enough of the substance to meet daily requirements.

Deficiencies

Rickets is the disease associated with vitamin D deficiency. This bone disease is caused by inadequate absorption of calcium and phosphate from the intestine. The resulting bone defects are caused by inadequate calcification secondary to an inadequate supply of calcium. The bones of patients with rickets become soft, and the stress and strain of weight bearing give rise to spinal and long-bone deformities. In adults, vitamin D deficiency results in osteomalacia, a disease characterized by a generalized decrease in bone density much like that seen in osteoporosis.

Toxicities

Hypervitaminosis D can lead to problems resulting from altered calcium metabolism. Again, such problems occur primarily in children who are given vitamin D in excess. Signs and symptoms of people suffering from hypervitaminosis D include increased serum calcium, loss of appetite, deposits of calcium in the kidneys and other soft tissues, weakness, fatigue, lassitude, nausea, vomiting, and diarrhea. Paradoxically, a generalized osteoporosis can result.

Although pregnant women require increased vitamin D, their ingestion of excessive amounts can be deleterious to the fetus. High calcium levels in the fetus can suppress the function of the parathyroid gland and result in hypocalcemia, tetany, and seizures after birth.

Medical Uses

Medical uses of vitamin D include the prevention or cure of rickets, and the treatment of hypoparathyroidism. Increased exposure to sunlight also aids in the resolution of these deficiency diseases.

VITAMIN E

Much remains to be learned about the essential roles, or lack thereof, of vitamin E in humans. Vitamin E includes a group of compounds called *tocopherols,* the major one of which is *alpha-tocopherol.* In animals, vitamin E deficiency produces abortion in the pregnant female and sterility in the male. A syndrome similar to muscular dystrophy also may develop in animals with vitamin E-deficient diets. We do not know the mechanisms through which these effects on reproduction and muscle are produced. Vitamin E is known to act as an antioxidant, however; that is, it is a substance essential in preventing destruction by oxygen of certain fats in cell membranes. Because of this antioxidant effect, vitamin E may contribute to the maintenance of cell-wall integrity, muscle metabolism, and pregnancy. Other functions and therapeutic applications are largely conjectural at present.

Requirement

The daily requirement of vitamin E in humans is not known, since definite deficiency diseases in humans have not been delineated. The recommended intake is about 10 IU for men, 5 IU for infants, and 15 IU for pregnant women.

Sources

Vitamin E is widely found in foodstuffs, especially in vegetable oils (particularly wheat germ oil), vegetables, fruits, grains, and dairy products.

Toxicities

A syndrome of clearly defined vitamin E toxicity has not been described, although dozens of alleged harmful effects resulting from high doses of vitamin E in humans have been reported. Marshall and Barrett (1985) discuss these reports.

Therapeutic Uses

The lack of vitamin E in human beings has been associated with various effects. Vitamin E supplementation has been attempted in the treatment of threatened abortion, recurrent abortion, male sterility, muscular dystrophy, cardiovascular diseases, and many disorders ranging from skin ailments to schizophrenia. In premature infants who need very high concentrations of oxygen, vitamin E has been administered to decrease the incidence of oxygen-induced eye damage (retrolental fibroplasia), although clear-cut evidence of its efficacy has not been given. Thus, because vitamin E has few clear-cut therapeutic indications and a low daily requirement, and because it is widely available in the diet, supplementation should not be necessary.

VITAMIN K

Vitamin K is essential for the normal biosynthesis of several factors required for the clotting of blood, the most important of which is the production of prothrombin by the liver.

Sources

Vitamin K is widely found in nature, and its highest concentrations are in leafy green vegetables, liver, grains, egg yolks, and dairy products.

Deficiencies

In the absence of vitamin K, prothrombin cannot be formed by the liver and the amount of clotting factors decline. This can result in spontaneous hemorrhaging. Deficiencies of the vitamin can result from inadequate intake and malabsorption, or as a consequence of the action of a vitamin K antagonist such as the anticoagulant drug *warfarin* (Coumadin) and its derivatives. Warfarin interferes with the biosynthesis in the liver of prothrombin and at least three other factors necessary for clotting. Administration of vitamin K can overcome this competitive antagonism and restore normal clotting.

Although it is unusual, malabsorption of vitamin K occasionally is seen in individuals with obstruction of the biliary tract, since the presence of bile in the intestine is required for the absorption of the vitamin.

Toxicities

Toxicities with vitamin K are rare, especially since this vitamin is seldom found in vitamin supplement preparations.

WATER-SOLUBLE VITAMINS

VITAMIN C

Vitamin C, in the form of limes, lemons, and oranges, has been used to prevent and treat scurvy since the mid-1500s. In about 1930, the antiscurvy substance in citrus fruits was identified as ascorbic acid (vitamin C), a six-carbon compound structurally related to glucose and other sugars (Figure 18.1).

FIGURE 18.1
Structural formulas of ascorbic acid (Vitamin C) and glucose.

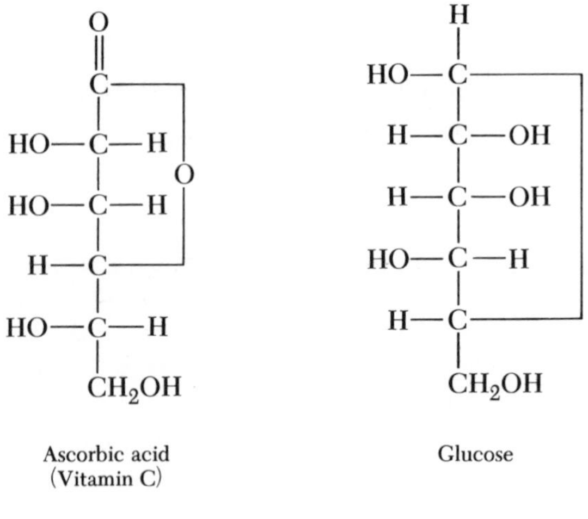

Ascorbic acid
(Vitamin C)

Glucose

Sources
Ascorbic acid is obtained from citrus fruits, tomatoes, strawberries, green vegetables, currants, and potatoes. Orange and lemon juices contain about 15 mg per ounce.

Requirement
The recommended daily requirement for vitamin C is 60 mg for adults, which increases during pregnancy and lactation. The body can store about 1500 mg of vitamin C; about 3 to 4 percent of this is used daily. Thus, 60 mg per day will maintain complete body saturation of the substance. One daily portion of a fresh food source of vitamin C usually will provide these quantities.

Deficiency
A deficiency in vitamin C intake can result in scurvy. Scurvy can occur in some elderly patients, alcoholics, drug addicts, and others with inadequate diets. Symptoms include weakness; small subcutaneous hemorrhages (petechiae); reduced wound healing; bleeding gums; bruises; thickened skin around hair follicles; and dryness of the skin, mouth, and eyes.

Biochemical Effects
Ascorbic acid functions in many biochemical reactions; it acts either as a coenzyme or as an antioxidant. The following appear to be necessary functions of vitamin C:

1. The normal synthesis of collagen and other connective tissues
2. The formation of normal teeth, bones, and blood capillaries
3. The synthesis of steroids in the adrenal cortex (see Chapter 14)
4. The synthesis of certain neurotransmitters
5. The ability to aid in wound healing and maintain the structure of blood capillaries and the gingiva by increasing collagen formation
6. The use of megadoses has been *postulated* to aid in treating a variety of illnesses ranging from the common cold to states of advanced cancer. These allegations remain unproved

Toxicities
Toxicity resulting from daily intake of 1 to 2000 mg is rare since much of the excess is excreted in the urine and feces. Continued use of megadoses (1 to 10 g per day), however, has been associated with the formation of kidney stones, rebound scurvy in newborns of mothers taking megadoses, and a similar rebound phenomenon in adults who cease such megadose therapy. These dosages are

totally unnecessary and risk the health of those who ingest them. Such levels should certainly be avoided in pregnant patients and in patients either with reduced renal function or a tendency to produce kidney stones.

Medical Uses

The only recognized therapeutic use for ascorbic acid is for the treatment of vitamin C deficiency, especially for the treatment of scurvy. Although megadose use probably is of no benefit in treating cancer or the common cold, the popular practice of taking 250 mg of ascorbic acid in the hope of reducing symptomatology should pose little or no risk.

THE B-COMPLEX VITAMINS

The "B complex" comprises many vitamins, all of which are involved in numerous metabolic activities. These vitamins, although separate types, usually are grouped together since they originally were isolated from the same common sources, notably liver and yeast. The B vitamins consist of eight recognized substances: thiamine (B_1), riboflavin (B_2), niacin (B_3), pyridoxine (B_6), cyanocobalamine (B_{12}), folic acid, biotin, and pantothenic acid (B_5). All are water soluble; excesses are excreted rapidly.

In addition to these eight compounds, several other substances have been alleged to be B vitamins, which are essential for health. Close examination has failed to reveal any essential role for these agents in human beings, however. Such compounds include choline (in egg yolk and fats), inositol (in fruits, plants, and cereals), para-amino-benzoic acid (PABA, a growth factor in bacteria), pangamic acid (B_{15}), and laetrile (B_{17}). Diseases caused by a deficiencies of these substances have not been reported, nor have the roles they play in human nutrition been defined. Other nonvitamins include carnitine (vitamin B_T), bioflavonoids (vitamin P), lecithin, rutin, vitamin Q, metanoic acid (vitamin U), and numerous others that occasionally are popularized with unsubstantiated claims from the health food industry.

Thiamine (Vitamin B_1)

All B-complex vitamins are essential as catalysts in various aspects of intermediary metabolism (Figure 18.2). Thiamine (as a pyrophosphate) functions in carbohydrate metabolism and is necessary for the breakdown of certain keto-acids into forms that can be used to produce energy. Thiamine is essential for normal neuromuscular

FIGURE 18.2
Some major metabolic pathways involving coenzymes formed from water-soluble vitamins. (From R. Marcus, and A. M. Coulston, "Water-Soluble Vitamins," in A. G. Gilman, L. S. Goodman, T. W. Rall, and F. Murad (eds.), *The Pharmacological Basis of Therapeutics*, 7th. ed. Macmillan, New York, 1985, p. 1552.)

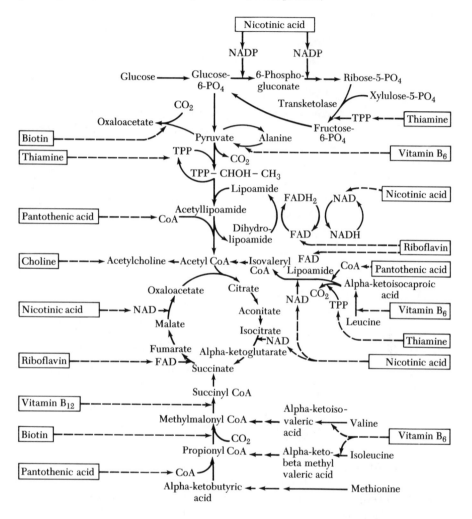

transmission and is involved in the synthesis of the transmitter acetylcholine. Thiamine also is involved in maintaining cardiac muscle tone, probably as an intermediary in energy production.

Sources. Foods rich in thiamine include pork, organ meats (kidney and liver), yeast, and grains. Many cereals and flour are enriched with thiamine.

Requirement. The recommended daily dose to avoid deficiency diseases is about 1.5 mg per day. Doses above about 5 mg per day are unnecessary since higher levels are poorly absorbed; even if they were absorbed, the excesses would be quickly excreted in the urine.

Deficiency. Beriberi, the disease associated with thiamine absence, involves dysfunction of the nervous and cardiovascular systems. Symptoms include impaired reflexes, altered sensation (pins-and-needles paresthesias), loss of muscle strength, cardiac palpitations, reduced cardiac output, and ECG abnormalities.

Toxicity. No major toxicities of thiamine have been reported, probably because excessive amounts are poorly absorbed and rapidly excreted.

Medical Uses. Thiamine is used most for the treatment of deficiency syndromes, especially those associated with nervous or cardiovascular symptoms. Malnourished individuals may require large daily doses (up to 40 mg) to delay or prevent the onset of serious neurologic, CNS, or cardiovascular consequences. At this stage, medical treatment is essential and self-medication may be dangerous.

Riboflavin (Vitamin B₂)
Riboflavin is essential for certain reactions of intermediary metabolism involving cellular respiratory and energy-producing processes.

Sources. Riboflavin is abundant in most dairy products, organ meats, and yeast. It also is present in enriched breads and cereals.

Deficiency. Signs of riboflavin deficiency include mouth lesions, dermatitis, anemia, neuropathies, corneal lesions, and cataracts.

Requirement. The recommended daily intake of riboflavin is about 1.3 to 1.7 mg. Excesses are excreted in the urine which can turn bright yellow in color. Patients with severe malnutrition may develop riboflavin deficiency and require aggressive therapy.

Toxicities. None reported.

Medical Uses. The only recognized use of riboflavin is in the treatment or prevention of riboflavin deficiency. In severely malnourished individuals or in patients on intravenous feedings for prolonged periods, riboflavin is included as part of an intravenous multivitamin replacement program. In such instances, the dose may be increased to 5 to 10 mg per day.

Niacin (Vitamin B₃, Nicotinic Acid, Nicotinamide)

Niacin is a coenzyme necessary for many metabolic processes essential for cellular energy production. Its role in the Krebs cycle is illustrated in Figure 18.2. The integrity of this process is essential for the biochemical conversion of carbohydrates, fats, and proteins into useable energy.

Sources. Niacin is readily obtained from liver, meat, poultry, fish, whole grains, and enriched breads and cereals. The amino acid tryptophane, found in milk and eggs, can be converted in the body into small amounts of niacin.

Requirement. The recommended daily intake of niacin to prevent deficiency is about 20 mg per day.

Deficiency. Lack of niacin in the diet leads to the clinical condition called *pellagra*. Characteristics of pellagra include diarrhea, dermatitis (mostly irritation of those parts of the skin exposed to sunlight), redness and swelling of the tongue, and dementia. Such deficiency commonly is seen in people suffering from chronic malnutrition and alcoholism.

Toxicities. Niacin may have some modest toxicities, but toxicity to the amide form, nicotinamide, is unreported. Niacin toxicities include itching, gastrointestinal distress, liver toxicity, and aggravation of peptic ulcers. Doses above the recommended daily requirement should not be taken by patients with liver disease, diabetes (niacin has an anti-insulin effect), or gouty arthritis (niacin increases uric acid levels in plasma).

Medical Uses. Niacin is used for the prevention and treatment of pellagra. Megadose levels of niacin have been used to lower blood cholesterol and to treat schizophrenia, but such uses probably are ineffective.

Pyridoxine (Vitamin B₆, Pyridoxal Phosphate, Pyridoxamine)

Pyridoxine is essential as a coenzyme for numerous reactions involving the metabolic utilization of amino acids, the synthesis of neurotransmitters, the formation of bile acids, and the development of the brain.

Sources. Pyridoxine is commonly found in meat, liver, fish, whole-grain cereals, and vegetables.

Requirement. The recommended daily requirement increases with the amount of protein in the diet; a dose of 2.0 to 2.2 mg per day usually is sufficient to handle a 100 g per day protein intake.

Deficiency. Pyridoxine deficiency is manifested as skin lesions, neuritis, anemias, and a variety of nervous system symptoms ranging from muscle weakness to convulsions. Again, toxicity is seen most in patients with chronic malnutrition and alcoholism.

Toxicity. The toxic potential of pyridoxine is low, but megadoses have been associated with sensory neuropathies, dependency, liver damage, and lethargy. Several important drug interactions involve pyridoxine. The effectiveness of L-dopa in treating Parkinson's disease, for example, is reduced, and B_6 should be avoided in patients receiving this drug. Blood levels of B_6 in patients taking isoniazid (see Chapter 20) and penicillamine (see Chapter 24) also are reduced, as these drugs increase the urinary excretion of B_6.

Medical Uses. A clearly defined deficiency syndrome has not been associated with pyridoxine. Patients with chronic malnutrition and lack of B-complex intake, however, can be presumed to have pyridoxine deficiency. The daily requirement is thought to be sufficient to meet any unrecognized deficiencies.

Cyanocobalamine (Vitamin B_{12}, Cobalamin)

When administered parenterally, vitamin B_{12} is curative for *pernicious anemia.* Vitamin B_{12} is not absorbed orally unless it combines with an "intrinsic factor" secreted by the stomach that is essential to the absorption of the vitamin.

Sources. To avoid pernicious anemia, human beings are dependent on dietary sources of Vitamin B_{12}. Large quantities of cyanocobalamine are found in meats, especially liver. Egg yolk and seafoods contain lesser amounts. The vitamin is absent in vegetable products, which places vegetarians at risk for developing deficiencies unless they take B_{12} supplements.

Deficiency. Lack of vitamin B_{12} results in disorders of the blood and nervous systems. Such disorders occur because vitamin B_{12} plays an essential role in DNA synthesis in dividing cells. Cells that demonstrate the most rapid rates of division show the most dramatic effects when the vitamin is absent. The red blood cells, which are especially sensitive, fail to mature when there is a B_{12} deficiency (because of decreased DNA synthesis) and die early; those that do survive are markedly abnormal. All other body cells are not so obviously affected because of their much slower rate of production and turnover.

Vitamin B_{12} deficiency also can result in irreversible damage to the nervous system. The myelin sheath of axons swells and dies; the death of the neuron itself follows. This results in sensory and motor losses followed by loss of memory and other cerebral cortical functions.

Requirements. The recommended dose of vitamin B_{12} to avoid pernicious anemia is 3 to 8 micrograms (μg) per day depending upon the person's age and sex. Excesses are excreted in the urine.

Toxicities. Cyanocobalamine is nontoxic to human beings.

Medical Uses. Vitamin B_{12} is prescribed for the blood and nervous system manifestations of pernicious anemia. In the absence of intrinsic factor secretion, B_{12} must be administered by injection. Tests of B_{12} in plasma combined with tests of gastric function will delineate the cause of pernicious anemia. Strict vegetarians or patients who have had their stomach surgically removed likely will require B_{12} supplementation. When any anemia is found, it should be carefully evaluated and multivitamin therapy witheld until a diagnosis is certain. The reason for this is that both B_{12} and folic acid (discussed next) will correct the blood component of pernicious anemia, but if lack of B_{12} is the culprit, the neurologic damage may go undetected until extensive, irreversible damage has occurred, because folic acid does not reverse the neurologic component. "Shotgun" use of vitamin B_{12} injections is considered poor medical practice if performed in the absence of diagnosed B_{12} deficiency. Vitamin B_{12} is *not* a health tonic; it is only a preventative for pernicious anemia. Elderly, ill patients with altered blood and neurologic function should be evaluated carefully for vitamin B_{12} deficiency.

Folic Acid (Pteroylglutamic Acid)
Folic acid is a coenzyme required for several biochemical reactions involving protein and nucleic acid synthesis. It is therefore required for blood cell production, the growth and development of body tissues, and the normal functioning of the CNS and GI tract.

Sources. Most foods are rich in folic acid, especially fresh green vegetables, liver, yeast, and beans.

Deficiency. Lack of folic acid produces an anemia identical to that produced by vitamin B_{12} deficiency. The nervous system is rarely, if ever, involved. Other symptoms of deficiency include weight loss, diarrhea, and sore tongue.

Requirement. The recommended daily intake of folic acid is 400 μg, even though only 50 to 250 μg usually is sufficient to cure the anemia.

Toxicity. There is none reported in human beings.

Uses. The therapeutic use of folic acid is limited to the prevention and treatment of folic acid deficiency. Accurate diagnosis is essential to differentiate folic acid deficiency from vitamin B_{12} deficiency as the cause of the anemia, since folic acid will resolve an anemia caused by a deficiency of either vitamin but it will leave the CNS component of pernicious anemia unchecked. Folic acid is therefore contraindicated in pernicious anemia and probably should be omitted from multivitamin preparations because it will obscure the diagnosis of unrecognized pernicious anemia.

Biotin
Biotin is a cofactor in carbohydrate and fat metabolism. As such, it is important in normal growth and the maintenance of nervous system tissue, skin, hair, muscle, bowel, and blood.

Deficiency. Deficiency of this element is characterized by neuromuscular disorders, severe skin irritation, loss of hair, muscle pain, lethargy, and depression.

Sources. Biotin is found widely in organ meats, egg yolk, peanuts, and some vegetables. Egg white contains none and, indeed, raw egg white contains a substance that binds to biotin with great affinity and prevents its absorption.

Requirement. The daily requirement of biotin in adults is 100 to 200 μg. Some biotin is manufactured by intestinal bacteria, and this is available for absorption.

Toxicity. None are reported in human beings, as excesses are readily excreted in urine and feces.

Pantothenic Acid (Vitamin B_5)
Pantothenic acid is required as a cofactor for several reactions involving the metabolism of carbohydrates, the synthesis of glucose, the synthesis and breakdown of fatty acids, and the synthesis of steroid hormones.

Sources. Pantothenic acid is widely found in organ meats, beef, egg yolk, bran, and peanuts.

Deficiency. Deficiency of pantothenic acid is associated with neuromuscular degeneration, adrenal cortical insufficiency, malaise, and infections.

Requirement. The required daily amount of pantothenic acid is about 4 to 7 mg, although dietary insufficiency is rare except in severe malnutrition because of its wide distribution in foodstuffs.

Toxicity. None reported in human beings.

Uses. No clearly defined syndrome of deficiency exists, but pantothenic acid is included in multivitamin preparations used for the treatment of severe malnutrition. Pantothenic acid deficiency is probably rare or nonexistent in individuals who eat a variety of foods.

READINGS

American Medical Association, "Vitamins and Minerals," in *AMA Drug Evaluations*, 6th ed., American Medical Association, Chicago, 1986, pp. 841–862.

Goodhart, R. S., and M. E. Shils (eds.), *Modern Nutrition in Health and Disease*, 6th ed., Lea & Febiger, Philadelphia, 1980.

Mandel, H. G., and V. H. Cohn, "Fat-Soluble Vitamins," in A. G. Gilman, L. S. Goodman, T. W. Rall, and F. Murad (eds.), *The Pharmacological Basis of Therapeutics*, 7th ed., Macmillan, New York, 1985, pp. 1573–1591.

Marcus, R., and A. M. Coulston, "The Vitamins: Introduction and Water-Soluble Vitamins," in A. G. Gilman, L. S. Goodman, T. W. Rall, and F. Murad (eds.), *The Pharmacological Basis of Therapeutics*, 7th ed., Macmillan, New York, 1985, pp. 1544–1572.

Marshall, C. W., "Vitamins and Minerals; Help or Harm?" Consumers Union, Mt. Vernon, NY, 1985.

Miller, D. R. and K. C. Hayes, "Vitamin Excess and Toxicity," in *Nutritional Toxicology*, vol. 1, Academic Press, New York, 1982, pp. 81–133.

CHEMOTHERAPY

CHAPTER 19

ANTIBIOTICS

Chemotherapy refers to the part of pharmacology that uses drugs therapeutically to destroy invading microorganisms while exerting little or no effect upon the host. The field of chemotherapy is concerned with many drugs, invading microorganisms, and infections caused by such organisms; the concept of chemotherapy has been expanded even further to include drugs used in the treatment of neoplasms, or cancers.

A *chemotherapeutic drug* is any drug used to destroy an invading, infecting organism or to treat cancer. An *antibiotic* is a chemotherapeutic drug that selectively destroys or inhibits the growth of invading bacteria, as opposed to viruses and fungi, etc. The original antibiotics used were produced naturally by various microorganisms found in soil samples; today, they may be obtained directly from cultures of such organisms, semisynthetically from natural substances, or totally by synthetic agents.

By definition, antibiotics exert a selective toxicity against invading bacteria and inhibit a process essential for their survival but not for that of the host, the person taking the antibiotic. *Bacteriostatic activity* refers to the ability of an antibiotic to *inhibit growth* of an organism; *bactericidal activity* refers to its ability to *kill* the bacteria (Figure 19.1). Antibiotics may be classified conveniently

---

FIGURE 19.1
Bacteriocidal or bacteriostatic effects of antibiotics on bacterial growth. Drugs are classified by their predominant effect at normal concentrations used clinically. (Modified from F. F. Cowan, *Pharmacology for the Dental Hygienist,* Lea & Febiger, Philadelphia, 1978.)

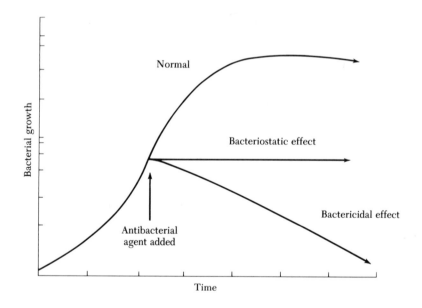

BACTERICIDAL ANTIBIOTICS	BACTERIOSTATIC ANTIBIOTICS
Penicillins	Sulfonamides
Cephalosporins	Tetracyclines
Aminoglycosides	Chloramphenicol
Polypeptide	Erythromycin
antibiotics	Lincomycin
Bacitracin	Clindamycin
Vancomycin	

as being of either type, although they are more frequently classified by their *chemical origin* and *spectrum of action*. When two bactericidal antibiotics exert a greater killing effect than either can singly, their effect is said to be *synergistic*. In contrast, when a bacteriostatic antibiotic reduces the killing effect of a bactericidal agent, such an effect is said to be *antagonistic*. Such considerations obviously govern drug selection when serious infections that require two or more drugs for eradication are being treated.

There are several mechanisms through which antibiotics exert their effects (Figure 19.2), including

1. Competitive antagonism with an essential substrate for bacterial growth (e.g., sulfonamides compete with para-amino-benzoic acid in the synthesis of folic acid in bacteria; bacteria synthesize

---

FIGURE 19.2
Sites and mechanisms of action of antibiotics. (Modified from F. F. Cowan, *Pharmacology for the Dental Hygienist,* Lea & Febiger, Philadelphia, 1978.)

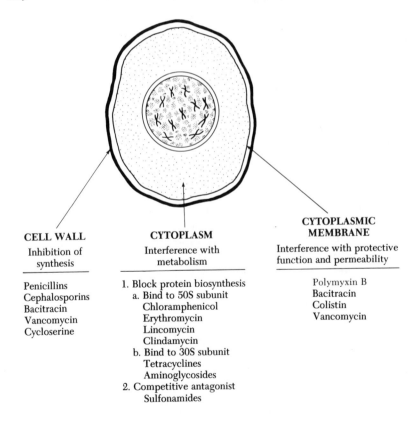

CELL WALL	**CYTOPLASM**	**CYTOPLASMIC MEMBRANE**
Inhibition of synthesis	Interference with metabolism	Interference with protective function and permeability
Penicillins	1. Block protein biosynthesis	Polymyxin B
Cephalosporins	a. Bind to 50S subunit	Bacitracin
Bacitracin	Chloramphenicol	Colistin
Vancomycin	Erythromycin	Vancomycin
Cycloserine	Lincomycin	
	Clindamycin	
	b. Bind to 30S subunit	
	Tetracyclines	
	Aminoglycosides	
	2. Competitive antagonist	
	Sulfonamides	

folic acid, but human beings cannot do so and must ingest folic acid as a vitamin)

2. Inhibition of cell wall synthesis (e.g., the penicillins and the cephalosporins)
3. A detergentlike action on cytoplasmic membranes that interferes with the protective and permeability characteristics of the membrane (e.g., polymyxin B and the antifungal agents)
4. Inhibition of cellular mechanisms for protein synthesis by binding to either the 50S subunit (e.g., erythromycin, chloramphenicol, lincomycin, and clindamycin) or the 30S subunit (e.g., aminoglycosides and tetracyclines) of the bacterial ribosomes

Of these mechanisms, two deserve special comment. First, bacterial cell walls are rigid, allowing bacteria to maintain a very high internal osmotic pressure. Blocking synthesis of this rigid wall leads to a protrusion of bacterial cellular contents, which ultimately leads to lysis and death of the cell. Second, many commonly used antibiotics—aminoglycosides, tetracyclines, chloramphenicol, lincomycin, clindamycin, and erythromycin—selectively inhibit protein synthesis in microorganisms. One of these, chloramphenicol, also inhibits protein synthesis in some host cells, which possibly accounts for some of the deleterious effects that limit its clinical use, despite its wide efficacy.

We turn now to the spectrum of actions of antibiotics—the range of effectiveness of given antibiotics against infections caused by various types of bacteria. For many years, bacteria have been divided into two groups according to their ability, or lack thereof, to be stained with a violet-colored dye. *Gram-positive bacteria* contain cell walls that have a permeability barrier to removal of the dye by an alcohol wash. *Gram-negative bacteria* have membranes that do not retain the violet dye when washed with alcohol. It is interesting to note that antibiotics frequently are differentiated by their ability to destroy selectively either gram-positive or gram-negative bacteria. Therefore, based on the Gram stain, bacteria have been divided into two groups: gram-positive (*Streptococcus*, *Staphylococcus*, and *Pneumococcus*) and gram-negative (*Neisseria*, *Pseudomonas*, *Proteus*, *Salmonella*, *Shigella*, *Escherichia*, and *Hemophilus*). Some antibiotics, such as many penicillins, have a narrow spectrum of action, while others, such as chloramphenicol and the tetracyclines, are effective against many organisms, although *no* antibiotic is universally effective against all microorganisms. In general, the narrower the spectrum of action, the more effective a drug is for an identified organism. Such an approach avoids problems associated with overgrowth of nonaffected organisms. Determining *sensitivity*, that is, testing an identified, infecting organism in culture with a variety of antibiotics, will identify those drugs to which the bacteria are sensitive. After determining sensitivity, choosing the drug with the narrowest spectrum of action makes therapeutic sense because the body's normal flora of bacteria will be least affected. Taking a broad-spectrum antibiotic in hopes of killing an unidentified pathogen and then hoping for the best is foolish, yet this is very frequently done. Such practice should be discouraged; it is wasteful and possibly harmful. Appendix III lists recommendations regarding specific antibiotics most useful for treating infections caused by specific microorganisms.

Problems associated with antibiotic therapy are many. First, large, walled-off abscesses usually are poorly penetrated by antibiotics and surgical drainage is necessary before effective antibiotic therapy can be initiated. Second, patients with depressed defense mechanisms (e.g., those with cancer or diabetes) are at increased risk of infection and may respond poorly to antibiotics. Third, bacteria can develop resistance to antibiotics to which they were previously sensitive. For example, some staphylococci, gonococci, and pneumococci produce the enzyme "penicillinase" that inactivates certain penicillins. This makes treatment of the diseases caused by these organisms much more difficult. Fourth, certain toxicities are associated with the use of antibiotics. Some produce specific damage, such as effects on the auditory nerve or the kidneys, and many, such as the penicillins, are capable of inducing an allergic response. This will be elaborated upon later when specific drugs are discussed.

SULFONAMIDES

The discovery of the antibacterial action of certain sulfonamides, as of sulfanilamide in the 1930s, marked a new era in the treatment of infection. Sulfonamides are antimetabolites in bacteria in that they prevent the synthesis of folic acid by a process of substrate competition.

Today, the use of sulfonamides is greatly reduced, primarily because of the introduction of other more effective, more specific antibiotics. However, sulfonamides are still widely used as bacteriostatic agents for the treatment of urinary tract infections and the prevention of infections in wounds caused by burns. Also, the recent development of a combination of a sulfonamide (sulfamethoxazole) plus another folic acid antimetabolite (trimethoprim) results in the sequential block of two steps in folic acid synthesis, which thus increases antibacterial effectiveness. This combination (marketed as Bactrim and Septra) is widely used in the treatment of several disorders, including urinary tract infections, bacterial bronchitis (caused by *Hemophilus influenzae* and *Streptococcus pneumoniae*), gonococcal genital infections (but not those caused by syphilis), and *Pneumocystis* infections in immunosuppressed patients.

Sulfonamides have a broad range of effectiveness against many gram-positive and gram-negative organisms, although for most systemic infections, the newer bactericidal antibiotics usually are preferred. Most sulfonamides have relatively short half-lives (about 4 to 7 hours), which necessitates that they be frequently administered to maintain therapeutic concentrations. Side effects include nausea, vomiting, loss of appetite, allergic reactions, and, rarely, serious liver, kidney, bone marrow, and blood cell toxicities.

For the treatment of urinary tract infections, most commonly caused by the gram-negative bacterium *Escherichia coli*, the sulfonamide sulfisoxazole (Gantrisin) usually is effective. For more resistant infections, however, the combination of sulfamethazole and trimethoprim may be needed. Sulfisoxazole occasionally is used to treat recurrent ear infections (otitis media) in children.

In severely burned patients, the topical application of sulfonamide *silver sulfadiazine* (Silvadene) prevents the growth of most bacteria and fungi. Its prophylactic use reduces bacterial infections of wounds from burns.

Sulfasalazine (Azulfidine) and several other sulfonamides are absorbed poorly from the GI tract, and because they concentrate in the bowel as a result, they are useful in treating inflammatory bowel diseases and for decreasing the intestinal bacterial flora.

Resistance. Bacteria may develop resistance to sulfonamides through poorly understood mechanisms, possibly those that involve increased substrate production that can overcome the competitive antagonism.

OTHER AGENTS FOR URINARY TRACT INFECTIONS

Several other antibacterial agents are used widely to treat urinary tract infections because of their effectiveness in the bladder against the gram-negative organisms that frequently cause such infections. Representative agents include nitrofurantoin (Furadantin, Macrodantin), methenamine (Mandelamine), and nalidixic acid (Neg-Gram). Nitrofurantoin is absorbed rapidly and excreted unchanged by the kidneys; thus, it concentrates in the bladder. In acidic urine, methenamine breaks down to liberate formaldehyde. Although nalidixic acid in the bladder selectively inhibits bacterial DNA synthesis, its use is limited by a narrow spectrum of action and by the rapid development of bacterial resistance.

PENICILLINS

Clinically, the penicillins are important, highly effective antibiotics of low toxicity. They presently are drugs of choice for the treatment of many infectious diseases. The mold *Penicillium chrysogenum* produces *penicillin G*, the only naturally produced penicillin used clinically. All other penicillins are semisynthetic derivatives of the basic penicillin nucleus obtained from fermentation.

As we discussed above, all penicillins inhibit cell wall formation in susceptible bacteria. The wall is composed of strands of aminosugars that are cross-linked by peptide (protein) chains. The penicillins block the formation of the cross-linked chains by binding to an enzyme, a *transpeptidase*, necessary for formation of the cross-linking. The lysis of the bacterial cell, and thus the bactericidal action of penicillin, follows from this effect.

Penicillin G (Table 19.1) is used widely in parenteral form primarily to treat infections caused by gram-positive organisms, including pneumococcal (e.g., pneumonia and meningitis), streptococcal (e.g., pharyngitis, pneumonia, otitis, sinusitis, meningitis, and endocarditis), meningococcal, gonococcal, and other organisms. Its use is limited by several important factors:

1. Penicillin G is poorly absorbed from the stomach and most is destroyed by gastric acids
2. It does not enter the cerebral spinal fluid (CSF) readily through the blood-brain barrier when the meninges are normal; when the meninges are inflamed, however, as in meningitis, CSF levels about 5 percent of plasma levels are obtained
3. It is rapidly excreted by the urine; its half-life is about 30 minutes
4. Most infections caused by staphylococci are resistant to penicillin G since these organisms have developed the ability to produce the enzyme penicillinase that destroys the penicillin
5. Many gonococci also have developed resistance to penicillin G, which necessitates higher doses to be given or a switch to be made to other antibiotics
6. Penicillin G is very allergenic; it produces a variety of reactions from rash to fatal anaphylaxis

TABLE 19.1
Spectrum of action of penicillins

Drug	Oral absorption	Penicillinase resistance	Dosage form	
			Oral	Parenteral
Penicillin G (Bicillin, Wycillin, others)	Poor	No	No	Yes
Penicillin V (PenVee K, V-Cillin K)	Good	No	Yes	No
Methicillin (Staphcillin)	Poor	Yes	No	Yes
Oxacillin (Prostaphlin, Bactocil)	Good	Yes	Yes	Yes
Cloxacillin (Tegopen)	Good	Yes	Yes	No
Dicloxacillin (Dynapen)	Good	Yes	Yes	No
Nafcillin (Nafein, Unipen)	Variable	Yes	Yes (not recommended)	Yes
Ampicillin (Amcill, Omnipen, Polycillin)	Good	No	Yes	Yes
Amoxicillin (Amoxil, Larotid)	Good	No	Yes	No
Carbenicillin (Geocillin)	None	No	No	Yes
Ticarcillin (Ticar)	None	No	No	Yes
Azlocillin (Azlin)	None	No	No	Yes
Mezlocillin (Mezlin)	None	No	No	Yes
Piperacillin (Pipracil)	None	No	No	Yes

Thus, with these limitations to penicillin G, other penicillins have been introduced to improve clinical utility.

Penicillin V has the same spectrum of activity as penicillin G, but it is much more stable in gastric acid and therefore much better absorbed when taken orally. It is widely available in tablets, drops, and suspensions. All other comments made for penicillin G apply to penicillin V.

There are five semisynthetic penicillins that are not destroyed by the penicillinase released by staphylococci and some gonococci. These drugs, therefore, are used primarily for infections known to be caused by these penicillinase-producing organisms. Available drugs in this category include *methicillin* (Staphcillin), *oxacillin* (Prostaphlin), *cloxacillin* (Cloxapen, Tegopen), *dicloxacillin* (Dycill, Dynapen, Veracillin), and *nafcillin* (Nafcin, Unipen). Of these, methicillin and nafcillin are absorbed poorly in oral form and are recommended primarily for parenteral use. The other three are acid stable and primarily administered orally.

Several penicillins have a spectrum of efficacy that is broader than that described above. The two major examples are *ampicillin* and *amoxicillin*. Both are well absorbed orally but are destroyed by penicillinase and therefore are ineffective against staphylococci. They are effective against various gram-positive and gram-negative organisms and are indicated therapeutically for the treatment of gonococcal urethritis, upper respiratory infections caused by *H. influenzae* and streptococci, and some cases of meningitis and *Salmonella* gastroenteritis.

Finally, several penicillins can be defined as "special purpose" or "antipseudomonas" in that they are used only in selected instances against infections caused by *Pseudomonas* or some *Proteus* species that are resistant to ampicillin and other penicillins. *Carbenicillin* (Geopen), *ticarcillin* (Ticar), *azlocillin* (Azlin), and *mezlocillin* (Mezlin) are examples. Since *Pseudomonas* and *Proteus* infections are serious and life-threatening, these drugs usually are given intravenously. Patients receiving them often are immunologically or otherwise compromised, which makes them at greater risk to the effects of infections. Obviously, these patients should be hospitalized and these drugs administered only in that setting.

CEPHALOSPORINS

The cephalosporins are a group of antibiotics first isolated from the mold *Cephalosporium acremonium*. Modern cephalosporins are semisynthetic derivatives of the original antibiotic. These agents inhibit bacterial cell wall synthesis in a manner similar to that of the penicillins. They differ from the penicillins in their antibacterial spectrum of effectiveness and in their resistance to penicillinase.

CLASSIFICATION

The ongoing development of newer cephalosporins with broader spectrums of action have necessitated a somewhat arbitrary classification by "generations" that is roughly based on antibacterial activity. The first-generation cephalosporins have an antibacterial spectrum similar to that of the penicillinase-resistant penicillins; that is, they are effective against gram-positive bacteria and only modestly active against gram-negative bacteria. The second-generation cephalosporins have an increased bactericidal activity against gram-negative organisms but one that is less effective than the extremely effective third-generation compounds. The latter compounds, however, are less active than the first-generation agents against gram-positive bacteria. Several cephalosporins penetrate into the CNS in sufficient concentration to be useful in the treatment of meningitis caused by gram-negative organisms. Moxalactam (Moxam) and cefotaxime (Claforan) are most effective in this regard.

The cephalosporins are excreted unchanged by the kidneys; renal failure prolongs their effectiveness. In patients with normal renal function, the cephalosporins' half-lives are two to four times longer than those of the penicillins.

ADVERSE REACTIONS

The cephalosporins share all of the toxicities of the penicillins. The most frequent side effect is an allergic reaction such as hives, bronchospasm, rash, serum sickness, and anaphylaxis. Since the cephalosporins and the penicillins structurally are quite similar, patients who are allergic to one agent may be allergic to all. (About 20 percent of penicillin-allergic patients may be allergic to cephalosporins.) Other toxicities have been reported, but their clinical importance is still being evaluated. Intolerance to alcohol (an Antabuse-like effect) has been reported with moxalactam, cefamandol, and cefoperazone.

USES AND MISUSES

The cephalosporins are used widely and probably are overused in situations in which other, less-expensive antibiotics with a more narrow spectrum are effective. They are, however, effectively used in the perisurgical period, for serious gram-negative meningitis, for upper respiratory tract infections caused by *H. influenzae*, and for the treatment of mixed infections of unknown organisms. As is the case with the use of all antibiotics, selection should be guided by identification and sensitivity testing of the microorganism.

OTHER INHIBITORS OF BACTERIAL CELL WALL SYNTHESIS

The penicillins and the cephalosporins are bactericidal because they inhibit the cross-linking reactions necessary for the formation of rigid cell walls in bacteria. Several other antibiotics act by inhibiting earlier steps in cell wall formation.

Cycloserine (Seromycin) is an orally administered, broad-spectrum antibiotic that competes with the amino acid alanine for an enzyme necessary in the formation of intermediates of larger proteins necessary for cell wall formation. Currently, cycloserine is used primarily in the treatment of tuberculosis, either as an adjuvant drug or when the bacillus is resistant to other drugs. CNS side effects limit the usefulness of the drug.

Bacitracin and *vancomycin* also inhibit intermediate steps in bacterial cell wall formation. Vancomycin is used intravenously to treat serious infections caused by staphylococci resistant to other drugs, especially in patients allergic to penicillin and the cephalosporins. Its half-life is about 6 hours. Its use is limited by auditory and kidney toxicities. Bacitracin is a broad-spectrum antibiotic primarily used topically in ointments and frequently in combination with other antibiotics (generally polymyxin B and neomycin) for treatment of superficial infections. Although it rarely causes allergic reactions when used topically, its clinical efficacy is dubious.

AMINOGLYCOSIDES

The aminoglycoside antibiotics are important drugs used to treat serious infections caused by gram-negative organisms. The mechanism behind their bactericidal action involves their interference with protein synthesis by their binding to protein subunits (the 30S ribosomal subunit). This action ultimately results in disruption of formation of cytoplasmic membranes located just inside the rigid bacterial cell wall. These drugs have several limitations:

1. They are poorly absorbed orally
2. They do not penetrate the blood-brain barrier into the CNS
3. They all are rapidly excreted by the kidneys
4. They produce serious toxicity, especially ototoxicity, involving both the auditory and the vestibular functions of the eighth cranial nerve, and nephrotoxicity; because these toxicities are related to blood levels of the drug, meticulous attention must be paid to drug concentrations in plasma and signs of toxicity carefully sought

Bacterial resistance may develop to these drugs. When widely used in hospitals to treat gram-negative infections, in fact, the emergence of resistant microorganisms can be a serious problem. Judicious use based on culture and sensitivity studies can reduce, but not eliminate, this problem.

Streptomycin, the oldest of the aminoglycosides (discovered in 1944), is used today primarily for treating tuberculosis and in combination with penicillin for treating bacterial endocarditis. It also is used to treat other rarer infections. Bacterial resistance develops rapidly.

Gentamicin, tobramycin, amikacin, kanamycin, and *neomycin* are used intravenously to treat serious life-threatening gram-negative infections. Neomycin also is available for topical and oral administration. Neomycin is not absorbed when administered orally; it remains in the intestine and greatly reduces the bacterial flora of the bowel. This action is useful both for preoperative preparation of patients for bowel surgery and for decreasing the production of urea and ammonia by intestinal bacteria in patients in states of hepatic coma (urea cannot be detoxified by the liver and contributes to the coma).

Amikacin has the broadest spectrum of antibiotic activity of the aminoglycosides; it is effective in patients who have developed resistance to other aminoglycosides. Such usefulness occurs because it is resistant to aminoglycoside-inactivating enzymes.

TETRACYCLINES

Development of the tetracycline antibiotics began in 1948 and continued until about 1970. They are recognized as the broadest of the broad-spectrum antibiotics and are useful against many gram-positive and negative bacteria as well as rickettsiae (e.g., Typhus and

Rocky Mountain spotted fever), chlamydia (e.g., urethritis), and mycoplasma (*Mycoplasma pneumonia*, Legionnaire's disease). Low doses are used widely to treat acne. Because of their broad spectrum, tetracyclines have been overused, and such use has led both to bacterial resistance in previously sensitive bacteria and to superinfections from organisms not sensitive to the drug. In general, these broad-spectrum, bacteriostatic agents are best replaced whenever possible by narrow-spectrum, bactericidal antibiotics for sensitive pathogens.

The tetracyclines act by inhibiting protein synthesis in bacteria (reversibly binding to the 30S ribosomal protein subunit). They are bacteriostatic rather than bactericidal.

Tetracyclines are variably absorbed when taken orally, ranging from 30 percent of the administered dose of chlortetracycline to 100 percent for minocycline. Calcium salts and gastric antacids bind tetracyclines in the stomach and prevent their absorption. Milk products and antacids should be avoided when taking tetracyclines. Tetracyclines have relatively long half-lives (about 8 hours), and high concentrations are found in bone, the liver, and the kidneys. They reliably cross both the blood-brain barrier and the placental barrier. Excretion is through the liver (in bile) and the kidneys.

Toxicities to tetracyclines are significant. Gastrointestinal side effects include nausea, vomiting, diarrhea, colitis, and bacterial, yeast, and fungal superinfections. Some host cells are affected by tetracyclines, and liver damage and an antianabolic action have been postulated. Tetracyclines can be deposited in developing teeth, with the risk being greatest between the neonatal period and about age 7 to 8 years. When taken during this time, teeth will develop a permanent brown discoloration. The intensity of discoloration appears to be dose-dependent. Tetracyclines also are deposited in the bony skeleton of the fetus, infants, and young children, which produces depression of bone growth. Thus, tetracyclines should be avoided in pregnant women and in children up to the age of 8 years. Other toxicities include photosensitivity of the skin and possible renal damage.

CHLORAMPHENICOL

Chloramphenicol (Chloromycetin) has a spectrum of activity that is similar to that of the tetracyclines. It interferes with protein synthesis by binding to the 50S subunit of bacteria and, to a lesser extent, by inhibiting mitochondrial protein synthesis in host cells, especially cells of the human bone marrow. The drug is mostly bacteriostatic. It is available for oral and intravenous use and is readily distributed throughout the body. (It has an excellent penetration into the CSF.) It is metabolized by the liver before excretion.

Despite excellent clinical efficacy, chloramphenicol's use is greatly restricted by the rare occurrence (about 1 : 10,000 to 1 : 30,000 patients) of severe, often fatal toxicities. The most important of these is irreversible depression of the bone marrow. Chloramphenicol should not be used in instances where other, less toxic antibiotics are effective; when it is used, its therapeutic advantages must be weighed against the risk of potential toxicity.

ERYTHROMYCIN

Erythromycin is used primarily to treat gram-positive bacteria that are resistant to penicillin. It also is extremely effective in treating *M. pneumoniae* infections, the pneumonia of Legionnaire's disease, and the genitourinary infections caused by chlamydiae, and in eliminating the carrier state for diphtheria. Erythromycin, like the tetracyclines, inhibits protein synthesis in bacteria, and its action is bacteriostatic.

Gastric secretions inactivate erythromycin, but enteric-coated tablets and salts of erythromycin are absorbed quite well. Such salts include erythromycin stearate (Ethril), erythromycin estolate (Ilosone), and erythromycin ethylsuccinate (E.E.S., Pediamycin).

Erythromycin concentrates in the liver and is excreted in bile. Very little is excreted in urine. Its half-life is 1.5 to 2 hours. Erythromycin does not diffuse into the CNS but does cross the placenta in significant amounts. It is one of the safest antibiotics available because allergic reactions to it are rare. A type of jaundice may occur, but, again, this is quite rare. The most common side effect is gastric upset.

LINCOMYCIN AND CLINDAMYCIN

Lincomycin (Lincocin) was isolated originally from soil collected near Lincoln, Nebraska. Its derivative, clindamycin (Cleocin), has replaced lincomycin in clinical use because of its increased activity and fewer side effects, although even the use of clindamycin is associated with significant toxicity (see the following paragraphs).

Available for oral or intravenous use, clindamycin inhibits protein synthesis in susceptible bacteria by binding to the ribosomes (again the 50S subunit) as does chloramphenicol. Its action usually is bacteriostatic, although it may be bactericidal in high doses. Its spectrum of action resembles that of erythromycin, and resistant strains of bacteria are common.

Clindamycin is well absorbed orally, has a half-life of about 3 hours, does not cross the blood-brain barrier in significant amounts, but does cross the placenta. The drug concentrates in bone, making it useful in treating osteomyelitis (infections of the bone). The drug is metabolized in the liver before its metabolites are excreted in urine and bile. Clindamycin exerts a powerful antimicrobial activity in the colon; this action accounts for its serious side effect. As colon bacteria are reduced, one resistant organism, *Clostridium difficile*, rapidly proliferates and secretes a toxin that can cause colon inflammation (colitis) that is characterized by diarrhea, abdominal pain, fever, and mucus and blood in the stools; it may cause fatalities. The first signs of diarrhea or abdominal pain during therapy necessitate that use of the drug be immediately discontinued. Use of narcotics to treat the symptoms of diarrhea or pain may worsen the condition and eventual outcome. Thus, while clindamycin is an effective antibiotic, it should not be used against infections that can be treated with other, less toxic drugs. Current clinical uses are limited to serious gram-negative infections, most often lung or abdominal abscesses caused by *Bacteroides fragilis*. Brain abscesses cannot be treated with clindamycin since it does not penetrate into the CSF.

Of interest is the recent observation that antibiotics other than clindmycin—ampicillin, for example—also may cause similar cases of antibiotic-associated colitis. Again, judicious use of any antibiotic is the best preventative of unwanted complications.

SPECTINOMYCIN

Spectinomycin is used intramuscularly for the treatment of penicillin-resistant strains of gonorrhea. Although it selectively inhibits protein synthesis in the organism, it is only bacteriostatic and many strains are resistant to it. It is not effective against other venereal infections such as syphilis or chlamydia.

POLYPEPTIDE ANTIBIOTICS

Certain antibiotics are polypeptides (proteins) that are isolated from cultures of bacteria. Such drugs include bacitracin, polymyxin B, colistin, and vancomycin. As a group, these drugs primarily are used topically, since they all have significant toxicity (especially to the kidneys) when used systemically. All four agents are bactericidal and inhibit cytoplasmic wall structure either by inhibiting its synthesis or by exerting a detergentlike action to disrupt a previously formed membrane.

Bacitracin, a mixture of several polypeptides, has an antibacterial spectrum similiar to that of the penicillinase-resistant penicillins. It is used topically to treat infections of the skin, conjunctiva, and the mucus membranes. Unlike penicillin, topical application of bacitracin seldom causes allergic reactions.

Polymyxin B is most effective when used topically against gram-negative bacteria. It is used to treat severe urinary tract infections (by transuretheral irrigation into the bladder), infected skin wounds, and infection of the external ear. Allergic reactions are rare.

Colistin has essentially the same activity, toxicity, and uses as polymyxin B.

Vancomycin (Vancocin), a toxic antibiotic that is bactericidal against gram-positive bacteria, prevents the formation of bacterial cell walls. Administered orally, it is poorly absorbed and excreted in the feces, which makes it useful in the treatment of severe cases of staphylococcal gastroenteritis and the colitis caused by the bacterium *Clostridium*. Administered intravenously, it is effective in treating serious infections caused by penicillinase-resistant staphylococci (*Staphylococcus pneumoniae* abscesses, endocarditis, and osteomyelitis), especially in patients resistant to the penicillins and cephalosporins. Toxicities include renal and auditory impairments and allergic reactions.

ANTIFUNGAL ANTIBIOTICS

Fungal infections can be classified conveniently as dermatologic, involving skin, hair, and nails; mucocutaneous, primarily *Candida* infections affecting moist skin or mucus membranes such as the oral cavity (thrush) or the vagina; or systemic.

Dermatologic fungal infections are treated topically with nonprescription drugs such as undecylenic acid (Desenex) and tolnaftate (Tinactin) or prescription drugs. More resistant infections of the hair or nails require prolonged oral administration of griseofulvin (Fulvicin, Grifulvin, Grisactin). Mucocutaneous *Candida* infections may be treated topically with amphotericin B (Fungizone), candicidin (Vanobid), nystatin (Mycostatin and others), clotrimazole (Mycolex-G), and miconazole (Monistat).

Systemic fungal infections are serious, chronic, and difficult to treat. Such infections often occur in patients with compromised defense mechanisms; the antifungal drugs can cause significant toxicity. The primary systemic agent is amphotericin B, although several other supplementary drugs also are available.

Griseofulvin is an antifungal agent that inhibits fungal mitosis by binding to intracellular proteins. When given orally for several months, it is incorporated into the skin, hair, and nails as well as into the fungus. Shampoos containing selenium sulfide (Selsun) are useful adjuvants. The half-life of griseofulvin is about 24 to 36 hours. Side effects are relatively infrequent, with headache and gastrointestinal upset being the most common.

Nystatin and *amphotericin B* both disrupt fungal membranes, altering their permeability and providing a fungistatic action. Amphotericin B, the primary drug for systemic fungal infections, frequently is lifesaving. It is used intravenously and its side effects, although significant, are more than offset by its efficacy against progressive, potentially fatal, fungal infections. When used topically for *Candida* infections, it is poorly absorbed and exerts little or no systemic effect.

Oral forms of nystatin are not absorbed and therefore are useful in treating fungal infections of the GI tract. It is too toxic for parenteral use. Used topically, it is effective against *Candida* infections that can be reached by topical application. Candicidin and miconazole are used in the treatment of vaginal *Candida* infections.

ANTIVIRAL AGENTS

The development of clinically effective antiviral agents is hindered by the fact that viruses are intracellular parasites that actually involve the host cells they invade. Drugs that injure a virus, therefore, also may injure the host cells harboring the virus. However, some recent advances have been made.

Idoxuridine (Herplex, Stoxil), which resembles the nucleic acid thymadine, is incorporated into viral and mammalian DNA and results in altered viral proteins due to faulty transcription. Topical use on the eye has proved effective in the treatment of herpes simplex-induced eye infections. Before this treatment was available, such infections frequently resulted in blindness.

Amantadine (Symmetrel) inhibits replication of influenza A viruses in humans, reducing the severity of the illness. It is well absorbed orally and is excreted unchanged in the urine. It is useful therapeutically as an alternative treatment to influenza vaccination (see Chapter 23) and to reduce symptoms after the infection has been contracted. It is also useful in the treatment of Parkinsonism.

Acyclovir (Zovirax) is particularly active against the herpes viruses since it interferes with DNA function. Herpes viruses exhibit a several hundredfold increase in toxicity to acyclovir compared to that for mammalian cells. Acyclovir is used to treat genital herpes, neonatal herpes, and herpes encephalitis. Other uses currently are under investigation.

Vidarabine (Vira-A), like idoxuridine, is effective topically against herpes simplex-induced conjuctivitis. It also is used in treating herpes simplex-induced encephalitis.

READINGS

American Medical Association, "Anti-infective Agents," in *AMA Drug Evaluations*, 6th ed., American Medical Association, Chicago, 1986, pp. 1225–1563.

"Chemotherapeutic Agents," in F. F. Cowan (ed.), *Pharmacology for the Dental Hygienist*, Lea & Febiger, Philadelphia, 1978.

Mandell, G. L., R. G. Douglas, Jr., and J. E. Bennett (eds.), *Principles and Practice of Infectious Diseases*, 2d ed., Wiley, New York, 1985.

Mandell, G. L., and M. A. Sande, "Chemotherapy of Microbial Diseases," in A. G. Gilman, L. S. Goodman, T. W. Rall, and F. Murad (eds.), *The Pharmacological Basis of Therapeutics*, 7th ed., Macmillan, New York, 1985, pp. 1066–1239.

Root, R. K., and M. A. Sande (eds.), *New Dimensions in Antimicrobial Therapy*, Churchill Livingstone, New York, 1984.

OTHER ANTI-INFECTIOUS AGENTS

DRUGS FOR MYCOBACTERIAL INFECTIONS

For centuries attempts to control tuberculosis and leprosy consisted of isolating the infected patient from the noninfected population. The introduction of antimycobacterial drugs has revolutionized treatment; most infected individuals can now remain in their community and lead productive lives.

TUBERCULOSIS

Tuberculosis still occurs frequently, but chemotherapy has provided effective methods of treatment. Such treatment destroys the bacillus (*Mycobacterium tuberculosis*), which reverses the symptoms and prevents transmission of the disease. Treatment is limited by several factors: (1) the slow rate of growth of the bacillus, (2) its protected location inside host cells, and (3) the fairly rapid development of tolerance of the organism to available drugs. These factors make prolonged drug therapy necessary. The three primary drugs used in treating tuberculosis are isoniazid (INH), ethambutol (Myambutol), and rifampin (Rifadin). Other secondary drugs are available, but because they usually are more toxic, they are used mainly in infections resistant to the primary drugs. Clinically, evident disease is treated with combinations of these three drugs; prophylactic therapy (as in a patient with a recent positive skin test) often consists of treatment with only a single drug (isoniazid).

Isoniazid is the single most effective drug for treating tuberculosis. It is extremely effective in killing the tubercle bacillus in concentrations that are relatively nontoxic to the host. It also is inexpensive, can be administered orally, and has a good patient acceptance. Isoniazid's mechanism of action likely involves the inhibition of mycolic acid biosynthesis, a necessary component of the mycobacterial wall. Since mycolic acids are specific to mycobacteria, such action explains the high degree of selectivity of isoniazid for mycobacteria. Isoniazid is distributed throughout the body, including the CNS, which makes it effective in the treatment of tuberculosis meningitis. Isoniazid is metabolized by a process called *acetylation*, the rate of which is genetically determined. Patients who are *slow acetylators*, about 50 percent of the U.S. population, demonstrate about a 3-hour half-life for the drug and high blood levels for a given dose. Patients who are *fast acetylators* demonstrate a 1-hour half-life for the drug and, in general, exhibit lower blood levels of the drug for the same dose. Accurate characterization of patients during therapy is important, as it affects both the effective dose and the toxicity.

Side effects of isoniazid are infrequent (occuring in about 5 percent of patients) and include rash, fever, peripheral neuritis, liver toxicity, arthritic reactions, and blood disorders. The peripheral neuritis is minimized by concurrent administration of vitamin B_6 (pyridoxine), 10 mg for every 100-mg dose of isoniazide.

Rifampin is the second most effective drug for treating tuberculosis and is used most often in combination with isoniazid. Also a broad-spectrum antibiotic, rifampin is effective against many gram-positive and gram-negative bacteria, although it is seldom used for anything other than tuberculosis. Rifampin acts by inhibiting RNA replication in mycobacteria and other organisms, thus blocking nucleic acid synthesis at concentrations lower than those at which it blocks RNA synthesis in mammalian cells. Rifampin is well absorbed orally; peaks at 2 hours; is widely distributed, including entry into the CNS; and is rapidly excreted in bile. The drug may turn body fluids (urine, sweat, and tears) an orange-red color. Side effects are infrequent and include rash, fever, nausea, vomiting, hepatic microsomal enzyme induction, and a potentiation of the hepatic toxicity of isoniazid.

Ethambutol is bacteriostatic to *Mycobacterium tuberculosis*; it interferes with protein synthesis by inhibiting the synthesis of its nucleic acids. Ethambutol is a useful adjunct to the bactericidal action of isoniazid and rifampin. It is well absorbed orally, penetrates poorly into the CSF, and is excreted unchanged by the kidneys. The only significant side effect of ethambutol is an optic neuritis, which can result in loss of visual acuity and the ability to differentiate red from green. This occurs in about 1 percent of patients, is correlated with the dose given, and is resolved by discontinuation of the drug.

LEPROSY

Although leprosy (Hansen's disease) is rarely seen in the United States and Europe, throughout the world (mostly in India, China, and Africa) about 12 to 20 million people have the disease. Leprosy is a mildly infectious disease caused by the bacillus *Mycobacterium leprae* (*M. leprae*). Most patients can be treated as outpatients because of the availability of effective chemotherapy and the relatively noninfectious nature of the disease. Five types of leprosy are described; effective treatment follows accurate classification. Multiple drug therapy generally is the treatment, just as it is for tuberculosis.

Dapsone (Avlosulfon) was the first effective modern drug against leprosy and it remains the mainstay of therapy. Another similiar drug is sulfoxone (Diasone). Both are taken orally, usually for several years. The most common side effect, lysis of red blood cells and other blood cell reactions, usually can be minimized by a reduction in the daily dosage. Expert medical guidance is essential for successful, safe treatment.

Other drugs effective against *M. leprae* include rifampin (discussed previously) and clofazimine (Lamprene). These usually are added to dapsone to provide coverage for dapsone-resistant strains of the bacillus. Clofazimine is a dye, and patients taking the drug may develop a red discoloration of the skin.

The national Hansen's disease center in Carville, Louisiana, provides consultation for physicians called upon to treat leprosy.

DRUGS FOR PROTOZOAL INFECTIONS

Protozoal infections are among the most common diseases in the world. Each class of protozoa contains organisms pathogenic for human beings. The *Sarcodina*, represented by *Entamoeba histolytica* (*E. histolytica*), cause amebic disentary; the *Mastigophora* (flagellates) cause trichomoniasis, giardiasis, and trypanosomiasis; the *Ciliophora* (ciliates) can infect man; and the *Sporozoa* cause malaria, toxoplasmosis, pneumocystosis, and other diseases.

Worldwide control of protozoa appears impractical and unobtainable. Immunization is unavailable. Chemotherapy is the only effective means of control. However, chemotherapy is expensive, frequently toxic, and unsuitable for wide use in countries with low standards of living and medical care. Environmental contamination, as in sewage, is a widespread reservoir of disease.

AMEBIASIS

Amebic dysentary is caused by *E. histolytica*. The disease has both intestinal and systemic components. Drugs used to treat the intestinal infection are those that are poorly absorbed from the intestine. Other drugs, metronidazole being the most effective, are used to treat both the intestinal component and the amebic infections of the liver and lungs.

Iodoquinol (Diodoquin), an important drug for treating intestinal amebic infections, often is combined with metronidazole. Other drugs used for intestinal infections include emetine (an alkaloid obtained from ipecac), the antibiotics tetracycline and paromomycin (Humatin), chloroquine, and certain arsenicals that now are considered to be obsolete.

Metronidazole (Flagyl) is an antibacterial agent useful in treating the systemic forms of amebic infections. It also has some intestinal activity. (For intestinal forms of infection it often is combined with iodoquinol.) Side effects are minimal and do not limit clinical use. When taken concomitantly with alcoholic beverages, however, metronidazole may cause a reaction like that caused by disulfuram (Antabuse). Metronidazole may be mutagenic, and its use in pregnancy is not recommended. Its possible carcinogenicity is being debated. Other uses of metronidazole include *Trichomonis vaginalis* infections, giardiasis, and certain systemic anaerobic (intestinal) bacterial infections.

Chloroquine (Aralen) is an antimalarial drug (see the following section) effective in treating amebic infections of the liver. It is less effective against intestinal infection.

MALARIA

Malaria is the single most common worldwide cause of suffering and death. Reductions in mosquito eradication programs and the appearance of strains of *Plasmodium falciparum* (*P. falciparum*) resistent to both insecticides and antimalarial drugs have resulted in recent resurgence of the disease. For centuries, malaria was treated with the bark of the cinchona tree, which contains quinine as the active antimalarial drug. Today, more effective drugs have been developed.

Classification of antimalarial drugs is complicated and is based on the life cycle of *P. falciparum*. Drugs that cure a clinical attack by eliminating the asexual forms of the parasite include chloroquine (Aralen), quinine sulfate, hydroxychloroquine (Plaquenil), and pyrimethamine (Daraprim). Tetracycline and combinations of a sulfonamide with the folic acid antagonist pyrimethamine also are effective. *Radical cure* is achieved by primaquine and implies the elimination of several forms of the parasite from the body. Specific drug therapy depends both upon the resistance to drugs of strains of *Plasmodium* in the area visited and upon the likelihood of exposure.

Clinical cure of chloroquine-sensitive strains of malaria usually can be achieved with a 3-day course of chloroquine. Quinine may be substituted when chloroquine-resistant strains of *Plasmodium* are present. Several drug combinations can be used for prophylaxis by visitors to endemic areas. Specific combinations to be used depend on the strains likely to be encountered.

Chloroquine is the drug of choice for treatment (clinical cure) of acute attacks of malaria in drug-sensitive strains of *Plasmodium*. It is rapidly absorbed orally and appears to be concentrated in the liver and the lungs. Side effects are low at moderate doses. The worldwide development of strains resistant to the drug is an increasing problem.

Quinine now is seldom used in treating malaria, except in combination with other drugs in chloroquine-resistant parasites.

Primaquine, as discussed previously, provides radical cure of most forms of the parasite. It is a poor suppressant of clinical attacks and is often combined with another drug to provide such coverage. It is rapidly absorbed orally and is rapidly metabolized and excreted. Side effects usually are mild except for a drug-induced hemolytic anemia (hemolysis of the red blood cells) that can occur in dark-skinned individuals. (Certain of these individuals have a genetic glucose-6-phosphate dehydrogenase enzyme deficiency that makes their red blood cells sensitive to primaquine and to several other drugs.)

Pyrimethamine and *trimethoprim,* both folic acid antagonists, inhibit the enzyme dihydrofolate reductase in malarial parasites. They are synergistic with sulfonamides (see Chapter 19) and often are used in combination with sulfonamides to treat malaria.

ANTHELMINTIC AGENTS

Drugs used to rid the body of parasitic worms (helminths) are called *anthelmintics,* whether the infection is in the intestine or is systemic with penetration into body tissues. It is estimated that over 2 billion people worldwide are hosts to helminths. Even highly developed countries have problems with helminths, especially with the advent of wide-ranging international travel.

Most parasitic worms enter the body through the mouth of the host, but some enter through the skin. Some, such as pinworms and whipworms, remain in the intestine; others lodge elsewhere in the body. Intestinal parasites usually are eradicated from the body easily and quickly with anthelmintic drugs, but systemic infections are difficult to treat. Effective treatment may be achieved only after identification of the infecting parasite. Submission of an appropriate specimen (stool, blood, sputum) to a parasitology laboratory often is necessary.

Infecting helminths may be roundworms (flukes) or flatworms (tapeworms). Anthelmintic drugs include

1. *Thiabendazole* (Mintezol), which is effective for strongyloidiasis and trichinosis
2. *Mebendazole* (Vermox), a broad-spectrum antihelminthic that is poorly absorbed orally and therefore useful against most intestinal infections (it is teratogenic in rats and therefore contraindicated in pregnancy)

3. *Pyrantel* (Antiminth), which is useful against all intestinal worms except *Trichuris* (it is a neuromuscular blocker in worms; it paralyzes them, weakens their grip on the intestinal wall, and allows them to be expelled in the feces)
4. *Piperazine* (Antepar), a drug similar to pyrantel but of second choice since some of it is absorbed and exerts a degree of toxicity to the host
5. *Diethylcarbamazine* (Hetrazan), a drug of choice for treating filariasis
6. *Niclosamide* (Niclocide), a drug of choice for treating tapeworm infections
7. *Praziquantel* (Biltricide), which is used for treating tapeworm infections resistant to niclosamide, and also for treating schistosome (blood fluke) infections which were formerly resistant to eradication
8. *Pyrvinium pamoate* (Povan), a cyanide dye useful in treating pinworm infections

R E A D I N G S

American Medical Association, "Anti-infective Agents," in *AMA Drug Evaluations*, 6th ed., American Medical Association, Chicago, 1986, pp. 1531–1613.

Mandell, G. L., R. G. Douglas, Jr., and J. E. Bennett (eds.), *Principles and Practice of Infectious Diseases*, 2d ed., Wiley, New York, 1985.

Mandell, G. L., and M. A. Sande, "Chemotherapy of Microbial Diseases," in A. G. Gilman, L. S., Goodman, T. W. Rall, and F. Murad (eds.), *The Pharmacological Basis of Therapeutics*, 7th ed., Macmillan, New York, 1985, pp. 1066–1239.

Root, R. K., and M. A. Sande (eds.), *New Dimensions in Antimicrobial Therapy*, Churchill Livingstone, New York, 1984.

CHAPTER 21

DRUGS USED TO TREAT CANCER

Recent years have seen significant advances in the chemotherapy of neoplastic diseases (cancers). Drugs may produce cures in patients with certain cancers, especially those involving white blood cells and the lymphatic system; when drugs have been combined with surgery and radiation therapy they have prolonged the lives of patients with many other forms of cancer. The design of more effective drugs used in various combinations based on the life cycle of cancer cells has led to improved therapeutic regimes. The cell life cycle can be briefly summarized as follows: (1) cells initially are in a resting phase that ends (2) with the sudden initiation of

FIGURE 21.1
Summary of the mechanisms and sites of action of anticancer drugs. (From P. Calabresi, and R. E. Parks, Jr., "Chemotherapy of Neoplastic Diseases: Introduction," in A. G. Gilman, L. S. Goodman, T. W. Rall, and F. Murad (eds.), *The Pharmacological Basis of Therapeutics*, 7th ed., Macmillan, New York, 1985, p. 1246.)

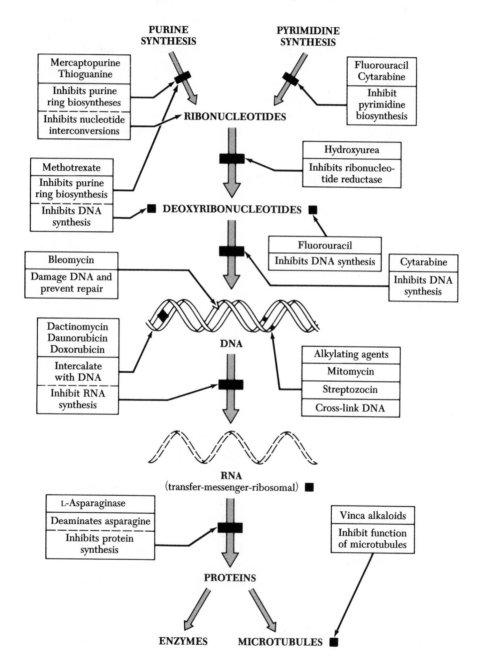

RNA synthesis, followed by (3) an increase in DNA synthesis that culminates (4) with mitotic division of the cell into two new cells.

Some antineoplastic drugs are specific for certain phases of the cell life cycle, while others are nonspecific. Most effective antineoplastic drugs act at specific phases of the cell life cycle and, therefore, are most effective against rapidly growing and dividing cells. Similarly, such drugs are most toxic against normal (noncancerous) body cells that normally grow and divide rapidly, such as cells of the bone marrow, hair follicles, and GI tract. Slowly growing tumors, such as colon and lung cancers, on the other hand, are less responsive to drug therapy.

The mechanisms of action of antineoplastic drugs are shown in Figure 21.1. Reference to the figure will be made as each class of drugs is discussed.

Drugs used in the management of cancers can be grouped conveniently into several categories:

1. Alkylating agents
2. Antimetabolites
3. Antibiotics
4. Hormones
5. Miscellaneous

Specific drugs within each category and the cancers against which each is most useful are listed in Appendix IV.

ALKYLATING AGENTS

The alkylating agents are highly reactive compounds that combine with various cellular components to form covalent linkages (alkylation). Such reactions are nonspecific for various stages of the cell life cycle, and the cytotoxic action of these drugs is thought to be secondary to alkylation of cellular DNA, especially guanine residues in the DNA. Side effects common to all these drugs include nausea, vomiting, bone marrow depression, and bleeding. Most of these agents have mutagenic and teratogenic potential and are cytotoxic to both cancerous and normal cells.

Four major types of alkylating agents are used therapeutically in cancer chemotherapy:

1. Nitrogen mustards
2. Alkyl sulfonates

3. Nitrosoureas
4. Triazines

NITROGEN MUSTARDS

The nitrogen mustards, discovered during World War II, were among the first anticancer drugs used. Representative nitrogen mustards include mechlorethamine (Mustargen), cyclophosphamide (Cytoxan), melphalan (Alkeran), and chlorambucil (Leukeran). These agents primarily are used in the treatment of Hodgkin's disease, lymphomas, multiple myeloma, and certain leukemias.

ALKYL SULFONATES

Busulfan (Myleran) is unique among the nitrogen mustards in that low doses exert a specific effect on a specific type of white blood cell called the granulocyte. Higher doses depress formation of other blood cells. Busulfan has little effect on lymphatic tissues and, therefore, is used mainly in the treatment of chronic granulocytic leukemias in which remission rates of about 90 percent are usually achieved.

NITROSOUREAS

The nitrosoureas available clinically include carmustine (BCNU), lomustine (CCNU), and semustine (methyl-CCNU). These agents all alkylate DNA and RNA. They are more lipid-soluble than other agents, which allows them to cross the blood-brain barrier and makes them useful in treating both primary and metastatic brain tumors. The limiting toxic effect is a profound, cumulative, and often delayed suppression of cell formation in the bone marrow. This toxicity is reflected by drastic reductions in white blood cell and platelet counts.

TRIAZENES

Dicarbazine (DTIC-Dome) markedly inhibits RNA protein synthesis. Like other alkylating agents, dicarbazine is cell cycle nonspecific. Its principal use is in treatment of malignant melanoma, for which it achieves a 20 percent overall success rate. Nausea, vomiting, and bone marrow depression are common toxicities.

ANTIMETABOLITES

An antimetabolite is a compound that bears close structural resemblance to a chemical used by the cell in essential metabolic processes. Replacement of a naturally occurring substrate with an antimetabolite disrupts important enzymatic reactions in the synthesis of nucleic acids, purines, and pyrimidines.

METHOTREXATE

Methotrexate (Folex, Mexate) (Figure 21.2) inhibits the formation of DNA and RNA by preventing the cellular synthesis of tetrahydrofolic acid. Methotrexate may produce striking remissions in acute leukemias in children. It also is used to treat lymphomas and, in women, choriocarcinomas and solid tumors of the breast, ovary,

FIGURE 21.2
Structural relationships between antimetabolic anticancer drugs.

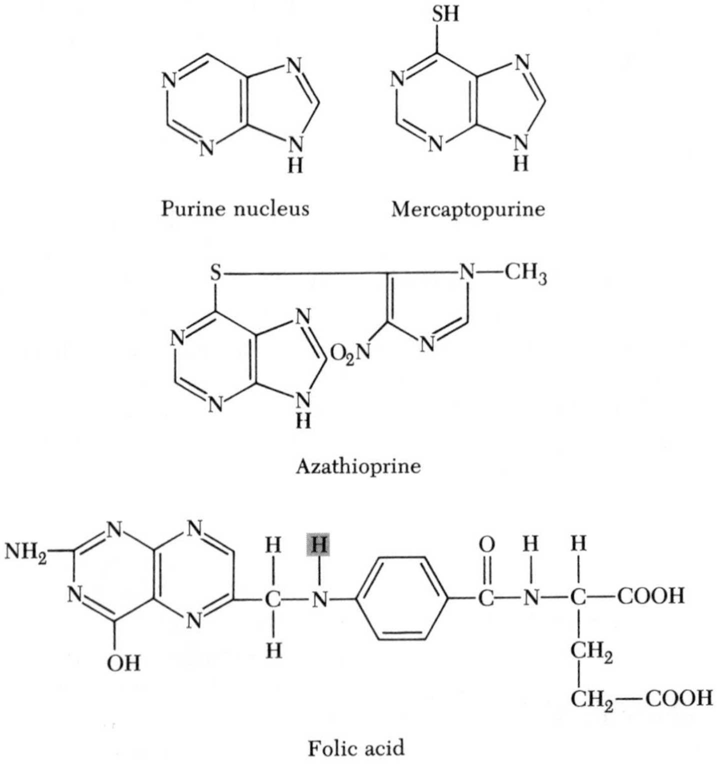

Purine nucleus   Mercaptopurine

Azathioprine

Folic acid

FIGURE 21.2 *(continued)*

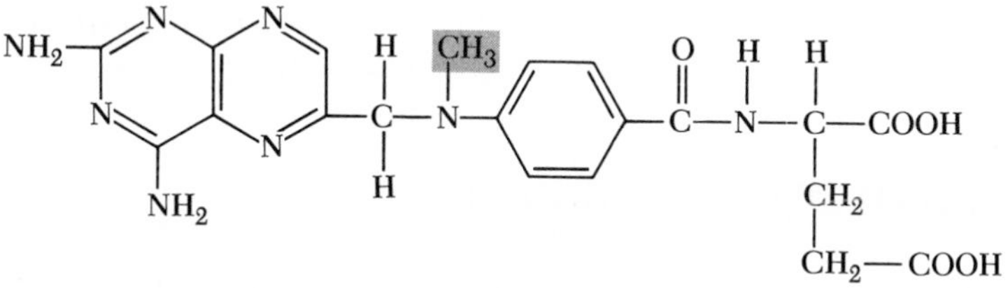

Methotrexate

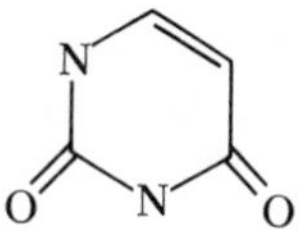

Pyrimidine nucleus 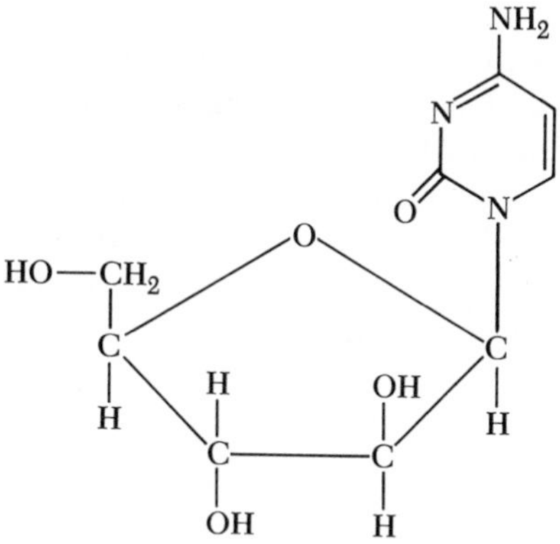   Cytarabine 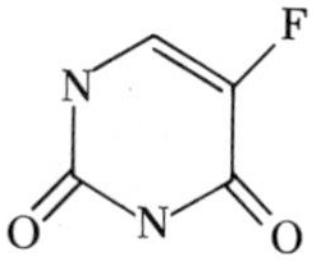   Fluorouracil

and colon. It is cell cycle specific, that is, it blocks the synthesis of DNA. Toxicities are many and include nausea, vomiting, diarrhea, loss of hair, rashes, ulcerations of the oral mucosa, and bone marrow depression. Rapidly proliferating tissues, such as hair, the mucus membranes of the GI tract and mouth, and the bone marrow, are most sensitive to cell cycle specific drugs.

PURINE ANTAGONISTS

Purine antagonists are used in medicine in many ways. Acyclovir and vidarabine are antiviral agents; azathioprine (Imuran) is an immunosuppressive used to prepare organ recipients for organ transplantation surgery; allopurinol is effective in the treatment of gouty arthritis; and *mercaptopurine* (Purinethol) and *thioguanine* are antitumor agents. These latter two drugs inhibit DNA and RNA synthesis through a complex series of steps (see Figure 21.1). Both drugs are effective in treating acute leukemias in children as well as other leukemias and lymphomas when combined with other drugs. They have little effect against solid tumors. Toxicities include bone marrow depression, nausea, vomiting, loss of appetite, and alterations in liver function. They are immunosuppressant, mutagenic, and possibly carcinogenic and embryotoxic.

PYRIMIDINE ANTAGONISTS

The major pyrimidine antagonists used as anticancer drugs are *fluorouracil* (5-FU) and *cytarabine* (Cytosar-U). Fluorouracil is useful in treating cancers of the colon, breast, ovary, pancreas, and liver by inhibiting RNA synthesis. (This inhibition is achieved by its competition with uracil for incorporation into RNA). It is cell cycle nonspecific and is usually used in combination with other antineoplastic drugs. Major toxicities are exerted on the GI tract and bone marrow. Cytarabine interferes with DNA synthesis by reducing the activity of the enzyme DNA-polymerase. Cytarabine is primarily used in the treatment of certain acute leukemias. Bone marrow depression is common.

ANTITUMOR ANTIBIOTICS

A number of antibiotics affect DNA synthesis or structure or interfere with RNA activity, which often leads to cellular destruction. *Bleomycin* (Blenoxane) causes DNA strand fragmentation and is useful clinically in treating testicular cancer, certain lymphomas, and squamous cell carcinomas of the head and neck. Bleomycin's most serious toxicity is its ability to cause fibrosis of the lungs in about 10 percent of the patients taking the drug. It causes little bone marrow depression.

Dactinomycin (Actinomycin D) combines with DNA and blocks RNA synthesis. When combined with other anticancer drugs, dactinomycin is useful in treating certain acute leukemias as well as several other cancers. It inhibits rapidly dividing cells of normal and cancerous origin. Thus, toxicities include all rapidly proliferating cells, which results in GI distress, loss of hair, bone marrow depression, and ulcerations of the oral mucosa.

Daunorubicin (Cerubidine) and *doxorubicin* (Adriamycin) are newer antitumor antibiotics; the former is used in acute leukemias and the latter in a variety of solid tumors. Aside from the usual toxicities associated with cytotoxic drugs, both can cause cardiomyopathy that can produce irreversible congestive heart failure. Other derivatives with less cardiac toxicity are being sought actively.

Mithramycin (Mithracin) is an antibiotic that binds tightly to DNA and inhibits RNA synthesis. Mithramycin is used clinically to treat testicular carcinomas. *Mitomycin* (Mutamycin) also binds to DNA and is used in the palliative treatment of various solid tumors. Both drugs are quite toxic.

HORMONES

Hormonal manipulation is useful in treating many types of tumors. Some tumors are *hormone-dependent* and regress when the hormone is removed by surgical excision of the structure producing the hormone. Removal of the ovaries, for example, may slow the growth of estrogen-dependent breast cancers. Castration is a treatment of choice for men with advanced cancer of the prostate gland. *Tamoxifen* (Nolvadex) is an antiestrogen that pharmacologically prevents estrogen stimulation of breast cancer cells, especially in postmenopausal women with estrogen receptor-positive advanced breast cancer (as determined by laboratory analysis).

Hormone-responsive tumors regress when high doses of certain steroid hormones are administered. Many tumors can be so classified and are affected by steroids (estrogens, androgens, progestins, and adrenal corticosteroids). Estrogens, such as diethylstilbestrol, are drugs of choice for the palliation of advanced carcinomas of the prostate gland. Similarly, progestins are effective in a palliative treatment of endometrial and ovarian cancers. Glucocorticoids, such as prednisone, may be cytotoxic in certain lymphomas and leukemias in children.

MISCELLANEOUS ANTITUMOR AGENTS

Streptozocin (Zanosar) is a naturally occurring nitrosourea antibiotic that both alkylates DNA and inhibits the synthesis of DNA. It is selectively taken up by the pancreas and is particularly useful in treating malignant tumors involving that structure. Kidney and liver toxicities are common.

The *vinca alkaloids, vinblastine* (Velban) and *vincristine* (Oncovin), are derived from the periwinkle plant. Both are cell cycle specific and block cellular mitosis, which inhibits cell division. Although structurally they are very similar, vinblastine and vincristine have some significant toxicologic differences. Vinblastine is a much more potent depressant of blood cell formation in the bone marrow (which limits its use), while vincristine causes a much greater loss of hair than does vinblastine. The clinical use of vincristine is often limited by neurologic toxicities that can be quite disturbing. Vinblastine frequently is used with other drugs in the treatment of metastatic testicular tumors as well as in Hodgkin's disease. Vincristine often is used with corticosteroids to produce remissions in certain childhood leukemias. Its mild degree of bone marrow depression makes it useful as an addition to other anticancer drugs in the treatment of a variety of cancers.

L-Asparaginase is an enzyme that catalyzes the conversion of asparagine to aspartic acid and ammonia. It was once thought that certain cancer cells required exogenous asparagine for growth while normal cells synthesized their own asparagine. This promise of an identifiable metabolic difference between malignant and normal cells has not been fulfilled, unfortunately, although combining L-asparaginase with other drugs has led to improved, although temporary, results in the treatment of certain leukemias. The drug is toxic to the liver, pancreas, CNS, and kidneys. Allergic reactions also are a significant problem.

Cisplatin (Platinol) is an inorganic platinum-containing compound that binds intracellular DNA and alters its geometry. Cisplatin is effective in the treatment of a number of cancers, including metastatic testicular and ovarian tumors. Its clinical utility is limited by kidney toxicity and damage to the auditory nerve.

Hydroxyurea (Hydrea) alters the synthesis of DNA and is useful in treating certain leukemias. Hydroxyurea is a potent bone marrow depressant, and this action underlies both its toxicity and its clinical utility.

Procarbazine (Matulane) is useful in treating Hodgkin's disease, presumably by blocking mitosis in both normal and cancerous cells.

Mitotane (Lysodren) is related to the insecticide DDT and is useful in treating certain tumors involving the adrenal glands. The mechanism of its specificity for the adrenals is unknown, but mitotane has little effect on the liver, the kidneys, or bone marrow. Since it destroys the adrenal glands, concomitant and subsequent use of glucocorticoids (see Chapter 14) usually is necessary.

READINGS

American Medical Association, "Drugs Used in Cancer Chemotherapy," in *AMA Drug Evaluations*, 6th ed., American Medical Association, Chicago, 1986, pp. 1167–1224.

Calabresi, P., and R. E. Parks, Jr., "Chemotherapy of Neoplastic Diseases," in A. G. Gilman, L. S. Goodman, T. W. Rall, and F. Murad (eds.), *The Pharmacological Basis of Therapeutics,* 7th ed. Macmillan, New York, 1985, pp. 1240–1306.

DRUGS AND IMMUNE MECHANISMS

CHAPTER 22

IMMUNOSUPPRESSANTS

Modulation of body immunity can be achieved by either of two means—the production of desired immunity or the elimination of undesired immune reactions. The former is achieved by either active or passive immunity; this is discussed in Chapter 23. The elimination of immune responses has become important in that it is used both to treat autoimmune diseases and to reduce the rejection of transplanted organs such as kidneys and hearts. Drugs used to achieve these ends are discussed in this chapter.

Lymphocytes are specialized white blood cells that provide, in large measure, for the body's defense mechanisms. There are two major types of lymphocytes, T and B; other types are being studied. T lymphocytes are manufactured at an early age in the thymus gland (hence, they are called T lymphocytes), and thereafter they circulate through lymph and vascular systems. They provide primary defense mechanisms against most viral, fungal, and protozoal infections, and many slow-onset bacterial infections, such as tuberculosis. They also play an important role in the body's vigilence against neoplastic cells, destroying those cells considered to be "foreign" to the body. In addition, T lymphocytes act to attract macrophage (phagocytic) cells to areas of inflammation or immunologic activity. They, therefore, regulate immunologic and inflammatory responses and react with substances recognized as foreign, such as inflammatory agents, tumors, and transplanted organs or grafts. Normal body tissues sometimes are mistaken for foreign material, that is, the system goes awry and the T lymphocytes attack normal tissues. Such diseases are termed "autoimmune" and include such syndromes as systemic lupus erythematosus (SLE), rheumatoid arthritis, myasthenia gravis, glomerulonephritis, hemolytic anemias, and thyroiditis.

B lymphocytes originally were thought to be produced in the bone marrow (hence, they are called B lymphocytes). These cells appear to have greater involvement in the production of antibodies against a variety of antigenic stimuli.

Several groups of drugs are used clinically to supress body immune responses, including

1. Corticosteroids, such as prednisone
2. Cytotoxic drugs
   A. Antimetabolites, such as azathioprine (Imuran)
   B. Alkylating agents, such as cyclophosphamide (Cytoxan)
   C. Folic acid antagonists, such as methotrexate
3. Immunosuppressents, such as cyclosporine (Sandimmune)

CORTICOSTEROIDS

Adrenal corticosteroids are widely used immunosuppressant agents that depress both immune and inflammatory responses. They have a wide margin of safety, reduce the rejection of donor organs, and often are used in combination with other immunosuppressants. The pharmacology of adrenal corticosteroids was covered in Chapter 14; included was a discussion of their anti-inflammatory action. Their immunosuppressant action is closely paralleled by their anti-inflammatory action—it is distinct from blockade of either histamine release or attachment of antigen with antibodies. Indeed, steroids such as prednisone do not inhibit these responses but appear to stabilize lysosomal membranes of lymphocyte cells and thus block the initiation or amplification of the immune response. They also appear to decrease the migration of T lymphocytes into areas of inflammation, which further decreases the intensity of the response. Clinically, use of corticosteroids produces best results in the autoimmune diseases.

Side effects of corticosteroids are the same as those discussed in Chapter 14 and include adrenal cortex suppression, a drug-induced Cushing's syndrome, and increased susceptibility to infections. Daily dosage may be needed during acute exacerbation of inflammation, but, when possible, dosage should be reduced and given on alternate days to minimize the adverse affects of continuous steroid therapy.

CYTOTOXIC DRUGS

Immunosuppression may be achieved with cytotoxic drugs (see Chapter 21), since they nonselectively destroy any rapidly reproducing cell, including the T lymphocytes that contribute to inflammatory responses. The primary impact of cytotoxic drugs occurs while antigens convert populations of B lymphocytes to cells that produce antibodies. This action produces an immune tolerance to specific antigens. Unfortunately, these cytotoxic drugs have such serious side effects as bone marrow depression (with loss of red and white blood cells as well as platelets), GI dysfunction, infections, and increased risk of both cancer and birth defects. These drugs were discussed at length in Chapter 21. Until recently, however, the combined use of cytotoxic drugs and adrenal corticosteroids were essential in establishing the feasibility of organ transplantation procedures, which decreased the likelihood of tissue rejection based on histoincompatability of the donor organ with the host cells. Newer advances hold promise for improved efficacy with decreased risk of toxicity.

CYCLOSPORINE

Cyclosporine is a unique immunosuppressant because it does not possess the overall cytotoxic actions of the drugs discussed above.

FIGURE 22.1
Chemical structure of cyclosporine.

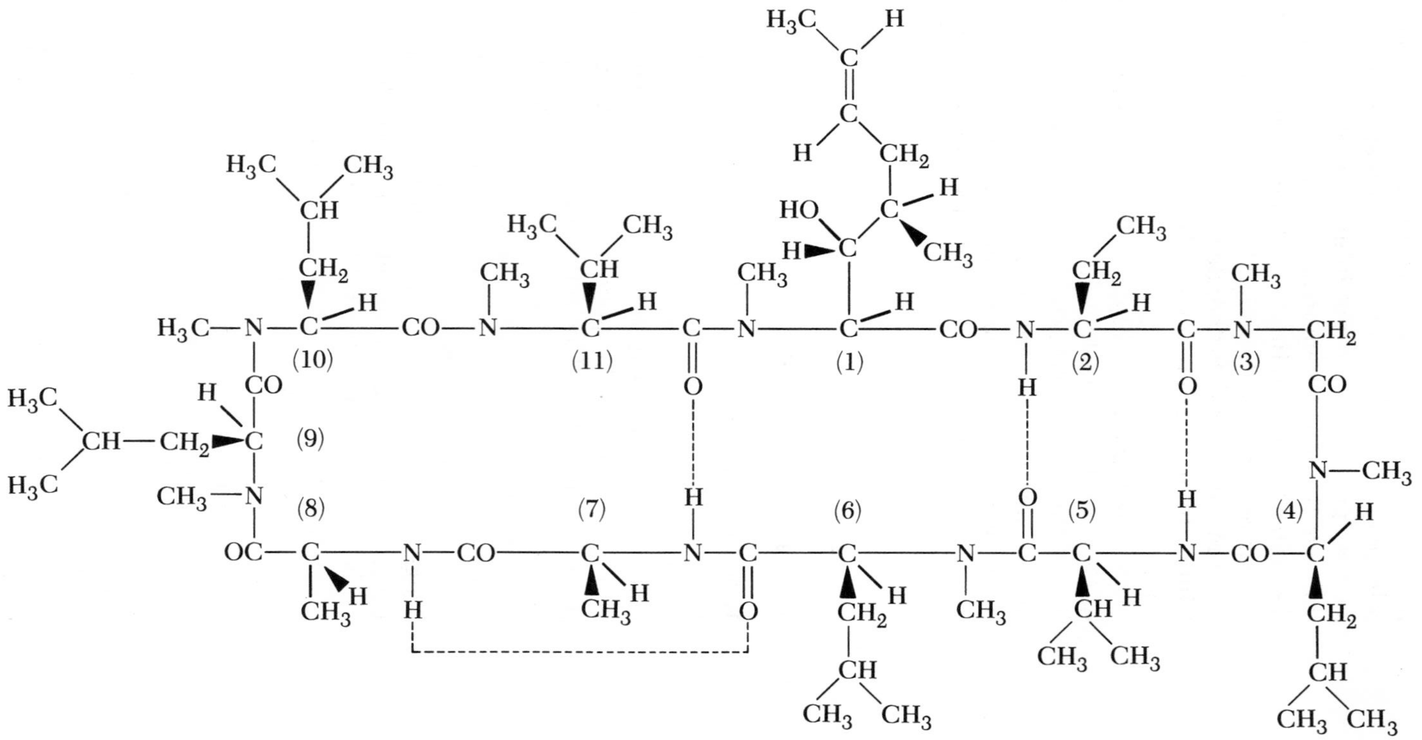

Cyclosporine is a complex molecule (Figure 22.1) produced by the fungus *Tolypocladium inflatum*. Cyclosporine specifically suppresses specialized cytotoxic T lymphocytes without decreasing the antibacterial or general cytotoxic defenses of the body. Nor does it decrease either the blood cell-producing functions of the bone marrow or the function of other white blood cells involved in body defenses, such as B lymphocytes. Cyclosporine appears to reduce the activation of T lymphocytes in response to foreign antigens, and it decreases other more complex steps in immunologic responses. Cyclosporine also appears to bind to and inactivate specific proteins (*cyclophilins*) in lymphoid tissue that appear to be crucial for the cytotoxic activation of T lymphocytes, although this is not yet fully clarified.

Cyclosporine is absorbed incompletely when administered orally; the intravenous dose being about one-third the oral dose. The drug appears to be bound to red blood cells, to plasma proteins, and to the cyclophilin proteins in lymphocytes. Cyclosporine is metabolized before excretion, although precise pathways have not been elucidated.

Therapeutically, cyclosporine is used as an immunosuppressant together with prednisone to increase the survival of the transplanted kidney, heart, liver, bone marrow, and pancreas. Its role in treating or ameliorating autoimmune diseases is being investigated.

As stated earlier, toxicities to rapidly proliferating cells have not been observed. Because some kidney and liver dysfunctions have been reported, these organs should be carefully monitored during therapy. Teratogenic, mutagenic, and carcinogenic effects appear to be much lower than those seen with the cytotoxic drugs, although one would expect that similar increases in susceptibility to infections would occur.

In summary, while the adrenal corticosteroids such as prednisone remain the mainstay of immunosuppression of autoimmune and transplant responses, the advent of cyclosporine provides additional hope for specificity of drug action with a minimization of generalized cytotoxic damage.

IMMUNOTOXINS

Although still in the experimental stage, the *immunotoxins* are composed of cytotoxic substances tightly bonded to antibodies which, in turn, bind the toxin to target antigens. The antibody binds to the antigen, which brings the cytotoxic substance into intimate contact with the antigen and allows for a more specific destructive effect. *Ricin* is a plant toxin that exerts its effect by blocking protein synthesis in those cells with which it comes into contact. Bonding ricin to antigen-specific antibodies allows it to exert a cytotoxic effect only on the antigen cells to which its antibody binds. Experimentally, ricin has had some success in killing certain animal tumors. The future of such products is filled with promise.

READINGS

American Medical Association, "Immunomodulators," in *AMA Drug Evaluations*, 6th ed., American Medical Association, Chicago, 1986, pp. 1147–1165.

Calabresi, P., and R. E. Parks, Jr., "Antiproliferative Agents and Drugs Used for Immunosuppression," in A. G. Gilman, L. S. Goodman, T. W. Rall, and F. Murad (eds.), *The Pharmacological Basis of Therapeutics*, 7th ed., Macmillan, New York, 1985, pp. 1247–1306.

CHAPTER 23

DRUGS USED
TO PRODUCE IMMUNITY

While the previous chapter focused on drugs that reduce the body's immunity in order to treat autoimmune diseases or to prevent rejection of transplanted organs, the present chapter discusses drugs that increase the body's immune defenses. This may be achieved either by administering preformed antibodies from another individual or species (*passive immunization*) or by administering an antigen that stimulates the body to produce its own antibodies (*active immunization*). Active immunization, achieved through innoculation with vaccines and toxoids, provides prolonged immunity. Passive immunization, using immune sera or antitoxins, is of short duration, usually only for the life span of the antibodies administered.

AGENTS FOR ACTIVE IMMUNIZATION

Drugs used for active immunization, that is, vaccines and toxoids, are specific antigens that induce the body to produce antibodies against infectious diseases. *Bacterial vaccines* are prepared from whole bacteria, (either killed or live, attenuated) that are not pathogenic in the form administered. *Toxoids* are detoxified byproducts of bacterial toxins from bacteria that induced disease primarily through the elaboration of an active toxin. Toxoids are not toxic, but they are antigenic, that is, they induce specific antibody formation. Bacterial vaccines and toxoids may be single agents (typhoid vaccine, tetanus toxoid) or combined (diphtheria and tetanus toxoids combined with pertussis vaccine). Viral vaccines are composed of live, attenuated viruses (measles) or killed viruses (influenza).

ROUTINE IMMUNIZATION

Immunization is recommended in childhood to provide active immunity against common infectious diseases, such as diphtheria, tetanus, and pertussis (caused by bacteria) and measles, rubella, mumps, and poliomyelitis (caused by viruses). The recommended immunization schedule is presented in Table 23.1. All of these immunizations are given by injection, except trivalent oral polio vaccine. Parents should keep an accurate record of immunization to insure that all doses have been administered. For children not immunized according to this schedule in infancy, physicians may use an alternative schedule and achieve satisfactory results.

VACCINES FOR SPECIAL SITUATIONS

BCG vaccine is a preparation of living BCG (Bacillus Calmette-Guerin) strain of attenuated bovine tuberculin bacillus used for active immunization against tuberculosis. This vaccine is not used routinely; it is only used for individuals with a negative tuberculosis skin test who are exposed repeatedly to patients with pulmonary

TABLE 23.1
Recommended immunization schedules for routine immunization

	2 mo	4 mo	6 mo	15 mo	18 mo	4–6 yr	14–16 yr
Diphtheria toxoid*†	✓	✓	✓		✓	✓	✓
Tetanus toxoid*†	✓	✓	✓		✓	✓	✓
Pertussis vaccine*	✓	✓	✓		✓	✓	
Trivalent oral polio vaccine	✓	✓	✓		✓	✓	
Measles vaccine‡				✓			
Rubella vaccine‡				✓			
Mumps vaccine‡				✓			

* Usually given as diphtheria and tetanus combined with pertussis vaccine (DPT).
† Tetanus and diphtheria toxoid boosters, given at 10-year intervals to maintain immunity.
‡ May be given as combined measles, mumps, and rubella (MMR) vaccines in a single dose.
SOURCE: Adapted from the American Academy of Pediatrics Committee on Infectious Diseases, 1982.

tuberculosis. Conversion to a positive skin test characterizes successful vaccination.

Cholera vaccine is a suspension of killed cholera organisms (*Vibrio cholerae*). Only short-lived immunization is produced, and even this occurs in only about one-half the patients receiving it. Because of this, vaccination is no longer required for travel to cholera-infected areas of the world.

Hepatitis B vaccine contains purified, noninfective hepatitis B surface antigens obtained from donors who are carriers of hepatitis B. Infectious potential is minimized both by treatment of the vaccine with formalin and by testing the vaccine in animals for lack of infectious potential. A series of three doses is given and at least 90 percent of recipients are immunized for at least 2 years. The vaccine is used in those at increased risk of contracting hepatitis B.

Influenza virus vaccine contains inactivated viruses of influenza strains predicted to be prevalent in the community in a given year. The vaccine is recommended for debilitated individuals, health-care workers, and adults over 65 years of age. Since the virus is cultured in chicken eggs, individuals allergic to eggs should not be vaccinated. The use of this vaccine has been associated with a rare neurologic syndrome called Guillain-Barre paralysis.

Other available vaccines include *plague vaccine* (a formaldehyde-killed preparation intended for individuals traveling to Cambodia and Laos), *pneumococcal vaccine* (for certain high-risk, immunosuppressed patients), *typhoid vaccine* (killed typhoid bacillus), *yellow fever vaccine* (live, attenuated virus), and *rabies vaccine* (killed virus) for individuals exposured to rabies.

AGENTS FOR PASSIVE IMMUNITY

Agents for passive immunity are called *antiserums* and contain antibodies produced in another individual. In contrast to active immunization, which induces antibody formation by the injection of bacterial or viral antigens, antiserums are active immediately, effective when no vaccine is available, and effective in individuals who are incapable of producing sufficient antibodies to protect them against exposure to an infecting agent. Most antiserums are used after exposure to an antigen. Antiserums of both human and equine origin are available; the latter is associated with a higher incidence of immediate allergic reaction and delayed serum sickness.

Hepatitis B immune globulin contains antibodies against the hepatitis B virus; it is obtained from human beings with high levels of such antibodies. The product is used to protect individuals exposed to hepatitis B and infants born to mothers with hepatitis B.

Immune serum globulin (gamma globulin) contains a pool of antibodies from normal donors. It is used most commonly to modify the measles response and to treat patients with certain antibody deficiency diseases.

Rabies immune globulin contains plasma proteins from donors with high levels of rabies antibodies. It is used for postexposure prophylaxis in patients known or suspected to have been exposed to rabies virus. It is commonly used in conjunction with rabies vaccine, although the globulin may prevent the production of active immunity by the vaccine.

Tetanus immune globulin contains antibodies from donors with high levels of such antibodies. It is used in patients with wounds contaminated by *Clostridium tetani* bacteria and for those who have not been adequately immunized with tetanus toxoid before exposure to the organism. The globulin is used together with antibiotic therapy. Similarily, active immunization with tetanus toxoid should occur concominantly with the use of the globulin.

Other agents used to provide passive immunity include *varicella-zoster immune globulin, vaccinia immune globulin,* and a variety of *antitoxins*. The latter are antibodies produced in horses. These antibodies combine with and neutralize harmful toxins released by animals (snakes) and spiders. These antitoxins, such as black widow spider antivenum, must be administered as soon as possible after innoculation with the toxin, as they do not reverse any tissue damage that occurs before the toxin is neutralized by the antitoxin.

R E A D I N G

American Medical Association, "Agents for Active and Passive Immunity," in *AMA Drug Evaluations*, 6th ed., American Medical Association, Chicago, 1986, pp. 1105–1146.

POISONS AND ANTIDOTES

CHAPTER 24

TREATMENT OF POISONING

The incidence of poisoning in the United States has been estimated to be about 1.7 million cases per year (Litovitz and Veltri, 1985). A single substance is implicated in 93 percent of poisonings. Oral ingestion accounts for 79 percent of poisonings; 90 percent of these are accidental, not intentional. Children account for about 70 percent of poisonings but only for about 7 percent of poisoning fatalities. Improved safety packaging of aspirin and prescription vials, along with increased parental awareness of the hazards of household chemicals, have contributed to a decrease in both the incidence and the severity of accidental poisoning in children.

At present, there are over 450 poison control centers in the United States; 34 regional centers have been designated by the American Association of Poison Control Centers. The location and telephone numbers of representative centers are listed in Appendix V. Information concerning the center nearest your home should be permanently displayed near all telephones.

PRINCIPLES OF TREATMENT

1. The diagnosis of poisoning is difficult. Physical signs may vary from unconsciousness to convulsions—CNS involvement is common (Table 24.1) and cardiovascular instability may be

TABLE 24.1
Signs and symptoms of CNS intoxication

Degree of severity	Characteristics
	Depressants
0	Asleep, but can be aroused and can answer questions
I	Semicomatose, withdraws from painful stimuli, reflexes intact
II	Comatose, does not withdraw from painful stimuli, no respiratory or circulatory depression, most reflexes intact
III	Comatose, most or all reflexes absent, but without depression of respiration or circulation
IV	Comatose, reflexes absent, respiratory depression with cyanosis or circulatory failure and shock, or both
	Stimulants
I	Restlessness, irritability, insomnia, tremor, hyperreflexia, sweating, mydriasis, flushing
II	Confusion, hyperactivity, hypertension, tachypnea, tachycardia, extrasystoles, sweating, mydriasis, flushing, mild hyperpyrexia
III	Delerium, mania, self-injury, marked hypertension, tachycardia, arrhythmias, hyperpyrexia
IV	As in III, plus convulsions, coma, and circulatory collapse

SOURCE: From C. D. Klaassen, "Principles of Toxicology," in A. G. Gilman, L. S. Goodman, T. W. Rall, and F. Murad (eds.), *The Pharmacological Basis of Therapeutics*, 7th ed., Macmillan, New York, 1985, p. 1599.

POISONS AND ANTIDOTES

present. Hysteria on the part of the discoverer of the patient may preclude rational reaction.

2. Appropriate reaction includes assessment of the poisoned individual, including his or her level of consciousness, respiratory adequacy, and presence of palpable pulses; identification of the poison ingested; and assessment of the surroundings in which the individual is found.

3. One must seek assistance immediately from professionals trained in handling crisis situations. This means that one should immediately contact both the nearest poison control center and the paramedics. (Usually, both contacts can be made through an emergency telephone operator.)

4. Overtreatment of a poisoned individual may cause more harm than good. One treats the patient and not the poison!

5. The mainstay of treatment is supportive care of vital organs. Assessment and maintenance of both respiration and circulation by basic cardiopulmonary resuscitation (CPR) techniques will prolong life until assistance arrives.

6. Early termination of exposure to the poison is essential for optimal treatment.

   A. *Topical exposure* to caustic chemicals necessitates prompt removal of all contaminated clothing and copious flushing with tapwater at low force. When the eyes are involved, flushing should be maintained for at least 15 to 20 minutes *by the clock*. When the skin or hair is involved, mild soap will aid in cleansing.

   B. When poisoning results from oral ingestion, emptying the stomach to prevent further absorption is essential and may be lifesaving. Indeed, induction of emesis is indicated after poisoning by oral ingestion of most drugs and chemicals. Exceptions include

      (1) Poisoning caused by the ingestion of strong acids or alkalis, such as lye and drain cleaners. These will cause even more damage to the esophagus when vomited.

      (2) Ingestion of certain petroleum distillates, such as kerosene, gasoline, and furniture polish. These may result in severe pulmonary damage if vomited and inhaled into the lungs.

      (3) Poisoning in patients who are unconscious, convulsing, in shock, and semicomatose, or in whom coma appears imminent. Such patients are at increased risk for aspiration of vomitus.

   The use of *ipecac* as an emetic is discussed in the following section. In the absence of ipecac, one should irritate the posterior pharynx (back of the throat) with the fingers, which may be sufficient to stimulate gagging and vomiting. Administration of activated charcoal to reduce absorption of nonvomited poison also is discussed later.

C. When overdosage results from parenteral injection of a drug, nothing can be done to prevent absorption. Hospital treatment will be aimed at supportive care, increased renal elimination of the drug (by manipulating urine pH, if possible or feasible), and the administration of any antidotes, if indicated.

7. In rare instances of poisoning, about 2 percent of cases, specific drug therapy may be considered to treat certain poisons. Available antidotes for these poisons are outlined below.

EMETIC DRUGS

Two agents available to stimulate emesis are *apomorphine* and ipecac. Apomorphine is seldom used today since it is not available in homes, must be given by injection, and causes CNS sedation and respiratory depression that occasionally require naloxone (Narcan) for reversal. However, apomorphine has a rapid onset (4 to 5 minutes) and is extremely effective in inducing regurgitation of gastric and upper intestinal contents. Its mechanism of action involves direct stimulation of the chemoreceptor trigger zone in the brainstem.

Ipecac syrup (dosage: 15 to 20 cm^3 in adults, 5 to 10 cm^3 in children less than 1 year of age) acts within 15 minutes; the dose may be repeated if emesis is not produced within that time. Failure of two doses to produce emesis indicates that gastric lavage (washout) should be performed by trained personnel. Ipecac syrup can be kept at home for emergency use, is inexpensive, and is quite safe. A glass of water administered after the ipecac syrup aids in inducing emesis. (*Caution:* Ipecac *extract* is 14 times more potent than ipecac syrup and must not be used because significant amounts may be absorbed; this can be toxic to the heart and even fatal.) But activated charcoal (discussed in the following section) should not be given concomitantly with ipecac syrup because it adsorbs the ipecac and nullifies its emetic effect. When given after the vomiting has ceased, the charcoal functions to adsorb any residual poison. Ipecac's mechanism of action involves local irritation of the GI tract. A 0.5- or 1-oz bottle of ipecac syrup should be kept in all homes with small children where accidental poisoning may occur.

CHEMICAL ADSORBANT

Activated charcoal, a potent absorbent for most poisons, acts by tightly adsorbing the poison to the surface of the charcoal particles. Since the charcoal particles are not absorbed from the stomach into the circulation, poison absorption is blocked, and the toxicity of the drug is greatly reduced. The poison–charcoal is excreted in feces. The surface area of 1 g of activated charcoal is over 3000 m^2. The recommended dose is 15 to 50 g (5 to 15 teaspoons in a glass of water). Again, the mixture is administered after emesis. Since activated charcoal absorbs any drug reaching the intestine, it also is useful in increasing the body's elimination of drugs such as tricyclic antidepressants, diazepam, and glutethimide that undergo enterohepatic circulation. Such drugs are secreted from bile into the intestine, are absorbed again, pass through the circulation into the liver, and eventually pass into the bile, and the cycle is repeated.

In past years, a "universal antidote" consisting of burnt toast, tannic acid, and magnesium oxide was advocated. The mixture of agents in the universal antidote tends to reduce the efficacy of the individual agents, and the pH of the antidote favors absorption of certain poisons. Today, this is discouraged in favor of the ipecac syrup–activated charcoal sequence.

SPECIFIC ANTIDOTES

Few specific drug or poison antidotes exist in medicine, but several of them that do exist and possess therapeutic use bear brief discussion.

1. *Heavy metal poisoning* is a serious industrial toxicologic problem. Terminating exposure is essential. In addition, certain drugs will inactivate absorbed metal ions. Agents utilized include
   A. *Dimercaprol* for mercury, gold, and arsenic poisoning.
   B. *Edetate calcium disodium* for lead poisoning.
   C. *Deferoxamine* for iron poisoning.
   D. *Penicillamine* (Cuprimine), an inactive degradation product of penicillin, for copper poisoning and poisoning by several other metals.
   These four agents chemically react with the metal ion and form water-soluble chelates that tend not to dissociate. This chelate complex is then excreted by the kidneys.

2. *Narcotic poisoning*, or overdosage, is characterized by severe respiratory depression and is treated by the intravenous administration of *naloxone* (Narcan), followed by use of respiratory support as necessary until the crisis has resolved.

3. *Acetaminophen (Tylenol) poisoning* may cause severe toxicity to the liver. *Acetylcysteine* (Mucomyst) inactivates toxic metabolities of acetaminophen and greatly reduces the incidence of liver toxicity. Thus, acetaminophen toxicity is treated by induction of emesis or gastric lavage, followed by doses of acetylcysteine at 4-hour intervals for several days, until such time as the total absorbed amount of acetaminophen is metabolized and the toxic potential is eliminated.

4. *Scopolamine* and *atropine poisoning* are treated specifically with drugs that inhibit the enzyme acetylcholine esterase. Such drugs increase total body acetylcholine and overcome the blockade of acetylcholine receptors produced by poisoning with these anticholinergic agents (see Chapter 3). Physostigmine (Antilirium), an example of such an acetylcholine esterase inhibitor, effectively antagonizes atropine and scopolamine poisoning.

5. *Cyanide poisoning* may result in severe tissue hypoxia. A cyanide antidote kit contains

   A. Amyl nitrite for inhalation.

   B. Amyl nitrite solution. (The nitrite reacts with hemoglobin to form methemoglobin. This, in turn, complexes with cyanide to form cyanomethemoglobin and preserves the integrity of cytochrome oxidase, an enzyme that otherwise would be bound and inactivated by the cyanide. The functional integrity of cytochrome oxidase is essential for preserving cellular respiratory capacity and thus oxygenation of body tissues.)

   C. Sodium thiosulfate to enhance the detoxification of cyanide to thiocyanate by liver enzymes.

6. Other specific antidotes are available for certain *insecticides*, such as the organophosphate acetylcholinesterase inhibitors, and certain *rodenticides*, such as those containing the anticoagulant *warfarin*. Hospital poison control centers are equipped to handle such emergencies with supportive therapy until specific treatment can be started.

7. Carbon monoxide (CO) poisoning results from inhalation of CO produced from incomplete combustion of organic chemicals such as gasoline. CO inhalation because of improper venting of automobile and furnace fumes causes many deaths each year. Toxicity results from the combination of CO with hemoglobin, which produces carboxyhemoglobin (COHb), a form of hemoglobin that does not carry oxygen to body tissues. Treatment of

CO poisoning is directed toward providing oxygen to the tissues and hastening elimination of the CO. Transferring the victim to fresh air is essential. CPR is needed if respiration has ceased. If poisoning is severe, treatment in a hyperbaric chamber is indicated. If this is unavailable, 100 percent oxygen should be given.

READINGS

Goldfrank, L. R., *Toxicologic Emergencies*, Appleton-Century-Crofts, New York, 1982.

Gosselin, R. E., R. P. Smith, and H. C. Hodge, *Clinical Toxicity of Commercial Products*, 5th ed., Williams & Wilkins, Baltimore, 1984.

Haddad, L. M., and J. F. Winchester (eds.), *Clinical Management of Poisoning and Drug Overdose*, Saunders, Philadelphia, 1983.

Klassen, C. D., "Toxicology," in A. G. Gilman, L. S. Goodman, T. W. Rall, and F. Murad (eds.), *The Pharmacological Basis of Therapeutics*, 7th ed., Macmillan, New York, 1985, pp. 1592–1650.

Klassen, C. D., M. O. Ambur, and J. Doull (eds.), *Casarett and Doull's Toxicology: The Basic Science of Poisons*, 3d ed., Macmillan, New York, 1985.

Litovitz, T., and J. C. Veltri, "1984 Annual Report of the American Association of Poison Control Centers National Data Collection System," *Amer. J. Emer. Med.*, 3:423–450 (1985).

S E C T I O N *EIGHT*

APPENDIXES

READINGS

TEXTBOOKS OF PHARMACOLOGY

Bevan, J. A., and J. H. Thompson, *Essentials of Pharmacology: Introduction to the Principles of Drug Action*, 3d ed., Lippincott, Philadelphia, 1983.

DiPalma, J. R., *Basic Pharmacology in Medicine*, McGraw-Hill, New York, 1982.

Gilman, A. G., L. S. Goodman, T. W. Rall, and F. Murad (eds.), *The Pharmacological Basis of Therapeutics*, 7th ed., Macmillan, New York, 1985.

Goth, A., *Medical Pharmacology*, 11th ed., Mosby, St. Louis, 1984.

Kalant, H., W. H. E. Roschlau, and E. M. Sellers, *Principles of Medical Pharmacology*, 4th ed., Oxford University Press, New York, 1985.

Levine, R. R., *Drug Actions and Reactions*, 3d ed., Little-Brown, Boston, 1983.

Modell, W., *Drugs of Choice 1984–1985*, Mosby, St. Louis, 1984.

GUIDES TO PRESCRIPTION AND NONPRESCRIPTION DRUGS

American Medical Association, *AMA Drug Evaluations*, 6th ed., American Medical Association, Chicago, 1986.

American Society of Hospital Pharmacists, *Consumer Drug Digest*, Facts on File, Inc., New York, 1982.

Benowicz, R. J., *Nonprescription Drugs and Their Side Effects*, 2d ed., Perigee Books, New York, 1983.

The Editors of Consumers Guide, *The New Prescription Drug Reference Guide*, Publications International, Skokie, IL, 1985.

Graedon, J., *The People's Pharmacy*, St. Martin's Press, New York, 1985.

Graedon, J., *The New People's Pharmacy*, Bantam, Toronto, 1985.

Long, J. W., *The Essential Guide to Prescription Drugs*, 4th ed., Harper & Row, New York, 1985.

Physicians' Desk Reference, 40th ed., Medical Economics, Oradell, NJ, 1986.

Physicians' Desk Reference for Nonprescription Drugs, 7th ed., Medical Economics, Oradell, NJ, 1986.

The United States Pharmacopial Convention, *The Physicians' and Pharmacists' Guide to Your Medicines*, Ballantine, New York, 1981.

Zimmerman, D. R., *The Essential Guide to Nonprescription Drugs*, Harper & Row, New York, 1983.

COUGH AND COLD MIXTURES

Modified with permission from *AMA Drug Evaluations*, 6th ed., American Medical Association, Chicago, 1986, pp. 385–390.
See Chapter 12 for pharmacologic discussion of the agents.

MIXTURES

Many of the preparations listed in this section appear to have been formulated for the symptomatic treatment of minor respiratory disorders rather than for specific relief of cough. Thus, in addition to an antitussive, these mixtures usually contain one or more ingredients classified as expectorants, one or more sympathomimetic agents as bronchodilators or nasal decongestants, and antihistamines. The effectiveness of these mixtures when compared to single-entity preparations is not known.

It is recognized that the use of single-entity preparations is preferred but, since many patients with cough have other symptoms such as those associated with the common cold, certain combination products may be useful and convenient. If a mixture is to be used, it should meet the following criteria: (1) that it contain no more than three active ingredients from different pharmacologic groups; (2) that each active ingredient be present in an effective and safe concentration and contribute to the treatment for which the product is used; (3) that such products be used only when multiple symptoms are present concurrently; (4) that the mixture be therapeutically rational for the type and severity of symptoms being treated; and (5) that the possible adverse reactions of the components be taken into consideration.

The following commonly used preparations are listed for information only; inclusion in the list does not indicate approval or recommendation for use.

ANTITUSSIVE MIXTURES CONTAINING CODEINE (ALL SCHEDULE V PREPARATIONS)

Actifed-C Expectorant (Burroughs Wellcome). Each 5 ml contains codeine phosphate (10 mg), guaifenesin (100 mg), pseudoephedrine hydrochloride (30 mg), and triprolidine hydrochloride (2 mg).

Ambenyl Expectorant (Marion). Each 5 ml of liquid contains codeine sulfate (10 mg), ammonium chloride (80 mg), bromodiphenhydramine hydrochloride (3.75 mg), diphenhydramine hydrochloride (8.75 mg), guaiacolsulfonate potassium (80 mg), menthol (0.5 mg), and alcohol (5 percent).

Calcidrine Syrup (Abbott). Each 5 ml of syrup contains codeine (8.4 mg), calcium iodide anhydrous (152 mg), and alcohol (6 percent).

Cheracol Cough Syrup (Upjohn). Each 5 ml contains codeine phosphate (10 mg), guaifenesin (100 mg), and alcohol (3 percent).

Dimetane Expectorant-DC (Robins). Each 5 ml contains codeine phosphate (10 mg), brompheniramine maleate (2 mg), guaifenesin (100 mg), phenylephrine hydrochloride (5 mg), phenylpropanolamine hydrochloride (5 mg), and alcohol (3.5 percent).

Naldecon-CX (Bristol). Each 5 ml of suspension contains codeine phosphate (10 mg), phenylpropanolamine hydrochloride (18 mg), and guaifenesin (200 mg).

Novahistine Expectorant (Merrell Dow). Each 5 ml contains codeine phosphate (10 mg), guaifenesin (100 mg), phenylpropanolamine hydrochloride (18.75 mg), and alcohol (7.5 percent).

Novahistine-DH (Merrell Dow). Each 5 ml of liquid contains codeine phosphate (10 mg), chlorpheniramine maleate (2 mg), phenylpropanolamine hydrochloride (18.75 mg), and alcohol (5 percent).

Nucofed (Beecham). Each capsule or 5 ml of syrup contains codeine phosphate (20 mg) and pseudoephedrine hydrochloride (60 mg).

Pediacof (Breon). Each 5 ml of syrup contains codeine phosphate (5 mg), chlorpheniramine maleate (0.75 mg), phenylephrine hydrochloride (2.5 mg), potassium iodide (75 mg), and alcohol (5 percent).

Phenergan Expectorant w/Codeine (Wyeth). Each 5 ml of expectorant contains codeine phosphate (10 mg), promethazine hydrochloride (5 mg), guaiacolsulfonate potassium (44 mg), citric acid (60 mg), sodium citrate (197 mg), and alcohol (7 percent).

Phenergan-VC w/Codeine (Wyeth). Each 5 ml of expectorant contains same formulation as *Phenergan w/Codeine* plus phenylephrine hydrochloride (5 mg).

ADDITIONAL ANTITUSSIVE MIXTURES

Conar (Beecham). Each 5 ml of oral suspension contains noscapine (15 mg) and phenylephrine hydrochloride (10 mg) (nonprescription).

Conar Expectorant (Beecham). Each 5 ml contains noscapine (15 mg), guaifenesin (100 mg), and phenylephrine hydrochloride (10 mg) (nonprescription).

Conar-A (Beecham). Each 5 ml of suspension contains noscapine (7.5 mg), acetaminophen (150 mg), guaifenesin (50 mg), and phenylephrine hydrochloride (5 mg) (nonprescription).

Rynatuss (Wallace). Each tablet contains carbetapentane tannate (60 mg), chlorpheniramine tannate (5 mg), ephedrine tannate (10 mg), and phenylephrine tannate (10 mg); each 5 ml of pediatric suspension contains carbetapentane tannate (30 mg), chlorpheniramine tannate (4 mg), ephedrine tannate (5 mg), and phenylephrine tannate (5 mg).

Tuss-Ornade (Smith Kline & French). Each capsule (timed-release) contains caramiphen edisylate (40 mg) and phenylpropanolamine hydrochloride (75 mg); each 5 ml of liquid contains caramiphen edisylate (6.7 mg), phenylpropanolamine hydrochloride (12.5 mg), and alcohol (5 percent).

MIXTURES CONTAINING GUAIFENESIN OR OTHER EXPECTORANTS

(See previous lists for other combination products containing guaifenesin.)

Brexin (Savage). Each capsule contains guaifenesin (100 mg), carbinoxamine maleate (4 mg), and pseudoephedrine hydrochloride (60 mg).

Congess SR (Fleming). Each capsule contains guaifenesin (250 mg) and pseudoephedrine hydrochloride (120 mg).

Dimetane Expectorant (Robins). Each 5 ml contains guaifenesin (100 mg), brompheniramine maleate (2 mg), phenylephrine hydrochloride (5 mg), phenylpropanolamine hydrochloride (5 mg), and alcohol (3.5 percent).

Phenergan Expectorant (Wyeth). Each 5 ml contains guaiacolsulfonate potassium (44 mg), promethazine hydrochloride (5 mg), citric acid (60 mg), sodium citrate (197 mg), and alcohol (7 percent).

Phenergan-VC Expectorant (Wyeth). Each 5 ml contains same formulation as *Phenergan Expectorant* plus phenylephrine hydrochloride (5 mg).

Polaramine Expectorant (Schering). Each 5 ml contains guaifenesin (100 mg), dexchlorpheniramine maleate (2 mg), pseudoephedrine sulfate (20 mg), and alcohol (7.2 percent).

Robitussin-AC (Robins). Each 5 ml of syrup contains codeine phosphate (10 mg), guaifenesin (100 mg), and alcohol (3.5 percent).

Robitussin-DAC (Robins). Each 5 ml of syrup contains codeine phosphate (10 mg), guaifenesin (100 mg), pseudoephedrine hydrochloride (30 mg), and alcohol (1.4 percent).

Robitussin-PE (Robins). Each 5 ml of liquid contains guaifenesin (100 mg), pseudoephedrine hydrochloride (30 mg), and alcohol (1.4 percent) (nonprescription).

Terpin Hydrate and Codeine Elixir (Various Manufacturers). Codeine, glycerin, and terpin hydrate.

Triaminic Expectorant (Dorsey). Each 5 ml contains guaifenesin (100 mg), phenylpropanolamine hydrochloride (12.5 mg), and alcohol (5 percent) (nonprescription).

Triaminic Expectorant w/Codeine (Dorsey). Each 5 ml contains codeine phosphate (10 mg), guaifenesin (100 mg), phenylpropanolamine hydrochloride (12.5 mg), and alcohol (5 percent).

Tussar-2, Tussar-SF (Armour). Each 5 ml of syrup contains codeine phosphate (10 mg), carbetapentane citrate (7.5 mg), chlorpheniramine maleate (2 mg), guaifenesin (50 mg), sodium citrate (130 mg), citric acid (20 mg), and alcohol (5 percent) (*Tussar-2*) or (12 percent) (*Tussar-SF*).

Tussi-Organidin (Wallace). Each 5 ml of elixir contains codeine phosphate (10 mg), chlorpheniramine maleate (2 mg), iodinated glycerol (30 mg), and alcohol (15 percent).

Voxin-PG (Norwich Eaton). Each tablet contains guaifenesin (400 mg) and phenylpropanolamine hydrochloride (75 mg).

Zephrex (Bock). Each tablet contains guaifenesin (400 mg) and pseudoephedrine hydrochloride (60 mg).

ANTITUSSIVE MIXTURES CONTAINING HYDROCODONE (ALL SCHEDULE III PREPARATIONS)

Hycodan (Endo). Each tablet or 5 ml of syrup contains hydrocodone bitartrate (5 mg) and homatropine methylbromide (1.5 mg).

Hycomine (Endo). Each 5 ml of syrup or 10 ml of pediatric syrup contains hydrocodone bitartrate (5 mg) and phenylpropanolamine hydrochloride (25 mg).

Hycotuss Expectorant (Endo). Each 5 ml contains hydrocodone bitartrate (5 mg), guaifenesin (100 mg), and alcohol (10 percent).

Tussend (Merrell Dow). Each tablet or 5 ml of liquid contains hydrocodone bitartrate (5 mg), pseudoephedrine hydrochloride (60 mg), and alcohol (5 percent) (liquid).

Tussend Expectorant (Merrell Dow). Each 5 ml of liquid contains same formulation as *Tussend* plus guaifenesin (200 mg) and alcohol (12.5 percent).

Tussionex (Pennwalt). Each capsule, tablet, or 5 ml of suspension contains hydrocodone (5 mg) and phenyltoloxamine as cationic exchange resin complexes (10 mg).

ANTITUSSIVE MIXTURES CONTAINING DEXTROMETHORPHAN

Anatuss (Mayrand). Each tablet contains dextromethorphan hydrobromide (10 mg), phenylpropanolamine hydrochloride (25 mg), phenylephrine hydrochloride (5 mg), chlorpheniramine maleate (2 mg), guaifenesin (50 mg), and acet-aminophen (300 mg).

Cerose-DM Expectorant (Ives). Each 5 ml contains dextromethorphan hydrobromide (10 mg), phenylephrine hydrochloride (5 mg), phenindamine tartrate (5 mg), guaiacolsulfonate potassium (86 mg), sodium citrate (195 mg), citric acid (65 mg), and alcohol (2.5 percent) (nonprescription).

Cheracol-D Cough Syrup (Upjohn). Each 5 ml of syrup contains dextromethorphan hydrobromide (10 mg), guaifenesin (100 mg), and alcohol (4.75 percent) (nonprescription).

Dimacol (Robins). Each capsule or 5 ml of liquid contains dextromethorphan hydrobromide (15 mg), pseudoephedrine hydrochloride (30 mg), guaifenesin (100 mg), and alcohol (4.75 percent) (liquid) (nonprescription).

Dorcol Pediatric Cough Syrup (Dorsey). Each 5 ml of syrup contains dextromethorphan hydrobromide (5 mg), guaifenesin (50 mg), phenylpropanolamine hydrochloride (6.25 mg), and alcohol (5 percent) (nonprescription).

Novahistine-DMX (Merrell Dow). Each 5 ml contains dextromethorphan hydrobromide (10 mg), pseudoephedrine hydrochloride (30 mg), guaifenesin (100 mg), and alcohol (10 percent) (nonprescription).

Robitussin-CF (Robins). Each 5 ml of liquid contains dextromethorphan hydrobromide (10 mg), guaifenesin (100 mg), phenylpropanolamine hydrochloride (12.5 mg), and alcohol (4.75 percent) (nonprescription).

Robitussin-DM (Robins). Each 5 ml of syrup contains dextromethorphan hydrobromide (15 mg), guaifenesin (100 mg), and alcohol (1.4 percent) (nonprescription).

Rondec-DM (Ross). Each 5 ml of syrup contains dextromethorphan hydrobromide (15 mg), carbinoxamine maleate (4 mg), pseudoephedrine hydrochloride (60 mg), and alcohol less than 0.6 percent; each milliliter of drops contains dextromethorphan hydrobromide (4 mg), carbinoxamine maleate (2 mg), pseudoephedrine hydrochloride (25 mg), and alcohol less than 0.6 percent.

Triaminicol Decongestant Cough Syrup (Dorsey). Each 5 ml contains dextromethorphan hydrobromide (15 mg), ammonium chloride (90 mg), pheniramine maleate (6.25 mg), phenylpropanolamine hydrochloride (12.5 mg), and pyrilamine maleate (6.25 mg) (nonprescription).

Tussagesic (Dorsey). Each 5 ml of suspension contains dextromethorphan hydrobromide (15 mg), acetaminophen (120 mg), pheniramine maleate (6.25 mg), phenylpropanolamine hydrochloride (12.5 mg), pyrilamine maleate (6.25 mg), and terpin hydrate (90 mg); each tablet (timed-release) contains dextromethorphan hydrobromide (30 mg), acetaminophen (325 mg), pheniramine maleate (12.5 mg), phenylpropanolamine hydrochloride (25 mg), pyrilamine maleate (12.5 mg), and terpin hydrate (180 mg) (both forms nonprescription).

Tussar-DM (Armour). Each 5 ml of syrup contains dextromethorphan hydrobromide (15 mg), chlorpheniramine maleate (2 mg), and phenylephrine hydrochloride (5 mg) (nonprescription).

Tussi-Organidin-DM (Wallace). Each 5 ml of liquid contains dextromethorphan hydrobromide (10 mg), iodinated glycerol (30 mg), chlorpheniramine maleate (2 mg), and alcohol (15 percent).

Composition of cold remedy preparations

Preparation	Decongestant†	Antihistamine†	Analgesic†	Miscellaneous†
Actifed (Burroughs Wellcome): tablets, syrup	Pseudoephedrine HCl, 60 mg (tablets), 30 mg (syrup)	Triprolidine HCl, 2.5 mg (tablets), 1.25 mg (syrup)		
*Comhist LA (Norwich-Eaton): capsules (timed-release)	Phenylephrine HCl, 20 mg	Phenyltoloxamine citrate, 50 mg; chlorpheniramine maleate, 4 mg		Atropine sulfate, 0.0242 mg
*Comtrex (Bristol-Myers): capsules, tablets, liquid	Phenylpropanolamine HCl, 12.5 mg (capsules, tablets), 4 mg (liquid)	Chlorpheniramine maleate, 1 mg (capsules, tablets), 0.333 mg (liquid)	Acetaminophen, 325 mg (capsules, tablets), 108 mg (liquid)	Dextromethorphan HBr, 10 mg (capsules, tablets), 1.6 mg (liquid); alcohol 20 percent (liquid)
*Contac (Menley & James): capsules (timed-release)	Phenylpropanolamine HCl, 75 mg	Chlorpheniramine maleate, 8 mg		
*Coricidin (Schering): tablets		Chlorpheniramine maleate, 2 mg	Aspirin, 325 mg	
*Coricidin D (Schering): tablets	Phenylpropanolamine HCl, 12.5 mg	Chlorpheniramine maleate, 2 mg	Aspirin, 325 mg	
*Coricidin Demilet (Schering): tablets	Phenylephrine HCl, 6.25 mg	Chlorpheniramine maleate, 1 mg	Aspirin, 80 mg	
*CoTylenol (McNeil): capsules, tablets	Pseudoephedrine HCl, 30 mg	Chlorpheniramine maleate, 2 mg	Acetaminophen, 325 mg	

* Nonprescription.
† Milligrams in solid dosage form or 5 ml of liquid (except drops).

258

Preparation	Decongestant†	Antihistamine†	Analgesic†	Miscellaneous†
Deconamine (Berlex): tablets, elixir, capsules (timed-release)	Pseudoephedrine HCl, 60 mg (tablets), 30 mg (elixir), 120 mg (capsules)	Chlorpheniramine maleate, 4 mg (tablets), 2 mg (elixir), 8 mg (capsules)		Alcohol 15 percent (elixir)
Dehist (O'Neal, Jones & Feldman): capsules	Phenylephrine HCl, 15 mg; phenylpropanolamine HCl, 30 mg	Chlorpheniramine maleate, 8 mg		
*Demazine (Schering): tablets (timed-release), syrup	Phenylephrine, 20 mg (tablets); phenylephrine HCl, 2.5 mg (syrup)	Chlorpheniramine maleate, 4 mg (tablets), 1 mg (syrup)		Alcohol 7.5 percent (syrup)
Dimetapp (Robins): elixir, tablets (timed-release)	Phenylephrine HCl, 5 mg (elixir), 15 mg (tablets); phenylpropanolamine HCl, 5 mg (elixir), 15 mg (tablets)	Brompheniramine maleate, 4 mg (elixir), 12 mg (tablets)		Alcohol 2.3 percent (elixir)
Disophrol (Schering): tablets, tablets (timed-release)	Pseudoephedrine sulfate, 60 mg (tablets), 120 mg (timed-release tablets)	Dexbrompheniramine maleate, 2 mg (tablets), 6 mg (timed-release tablets)		
*Dristan (Whitehall): capsules, tablets	Phenylephrine HCl, 12.5 mg (capsules), 5 mg (tablets)	Chlorpheniramine maleate, 2 mg	Aspirin, 325 mg	Caffeine, 16.2 mg

* Nonprescription.
† Milligrams in solid dosage form or 5 ml of liquid (except drops).

(continued)

Composition of cold remedy preparations (*continued*)

Preparation	Decongestant†	Antihistamine†	Analgesic†	Miscellaneous†
*Dristan-AF (Whitehall): tablets	Phenylephrine HCl, 5 mg	Chlorpheniramine maleate, 2 mg	Acetaminophen, 325 mg	Caffeine, 16.2 mg
Drixoral (Schering): tablets (timed-release)	Pseudoephedrine sulfate, 120 mg	Dexbrompheniramine maleate, 6 mg		
*Entex (Norwich-Eaton): capsules, liquid	Phenylephrine HCl, 5 mg; phenylpropanolamine HCl, 45 mg (capsules), 20 mg (liquid)			Guaifenesin, 200 mg (capsules), 100 mg (liquid); alcohol 5 percent (liquid)
*Fedahist (Rorer): tablets capsules (timed-release), syrup	Pseudoephedrine HCl, 60 mg (tablets), 65 mg (capsules), 30 mg (syrup)	Chlorpheniramine maleate, 4 mg (tablets), 10 mg (capsules), 2 mg (syrup)		
Histalet (Reid-Provident): syrup	Pseudoephedrine HCl, 45 mg	Chlorpheniramine maleate, 3 mg		
Isoclor (American Critical Care): tablets, liquid, capsules (timed-release)	Pseudoephedrine HCl, 60 mg (tablets), 30 mg (liquid), 120 mg (capsules)	Chlorpheniramine maleate, 4 mg (tablets), 2 mg (liquid), 8 mg (capsules)		
Naldecon (Bristol): syrup, tablets (timed-release)	Phenylpropanolamine HCl, 40 mg (tablets), 20 mg (syrup); phenylephrine HCl, 10 mg (tablets), 5 mg (syrup)	Phenyltoloxamine citrate, 15 mg (tablets), 7.5 mg (syrup); chlorpheniramine maleate, 5 mg (tablets), 2.5 mg (syrup)		
Nolamine (Carnrick): tablets (timed-release)	Phenylpropanolamine HCl, 50 mg	Chlorpheniramine maleate, 4 mg; phenindamine tartrate, 24 mg		

* Nonprescription.

Preparation	Decongestant†	Antihistamine†	Analgesic†	Miscellaneous†
Novafed A (Merrell Dow): capsules (timed-release), liquid	Pseudoephedrine HCl, 120 mg (capsules), 30 mg (liquid)	Chlorpheniramine maleate, 8 mg (capsules), 2 mg (liquid)		Alcohol 5 percent (liquid)
*Novahistine Elixir (Merrell Dow): elixir	Phenylpropanolamine, 18.5 mg	Chlorpheniramine maleate, 2 mg		Alcohol 5 percent
Ornade (Smith Kline & French): capsules (timed-release)	Phenylpropanolamine HCl, 75 mg	Chlorpheniramine maleate, 12 mg		
Rondec (Ross): drops, syrup, tablets	Pseudoephedrine HCl, 25 mg/ml (drops), 60 mg (syrup, tablets)	Carbinoxamine maleate, 2 mg/ml (drops), 4 mg (syrup, tablets)		
Rynatan (Wallace): tablets	Phenylephrine tannate, 25 mg	Chlorpheniramine tannate, 8 mg; pyrilamine tannate, 25 mg		
Singlet (Merrell Dow): tablets (timed-release)	Phenylephrine HCl, 40 mg	Chlorpheniramine maleate, 8 mg	Acetaminophen, 500 mg	
Sinubid (Parke, Davis): tablets	Phenylpropanolamine HCl, 100 mg	Phenyltoloxamine citrate, 66 mg	Acetaminophen, 300 mg; phenacetin, 300 mg	
*Sinulin (Carnrick): tablets	Phenylpropanolamine HCl, 37.5 mg	Chlorpheniramine maleate, 2 mg	Acetaminophen, 325 mg; salicylamide, 250 mg	Homatropine methylbromide, 0.75 mg

* Nonprescription.
† Milligrams in solid dosage form or 5 ml of liquid (except drops).

(*continued*)

Composition of cold remedy preparations *(continued)*

Preparation	Decongestant[†]	Antihistamine[†]	Analgesic[†]	Miscellaneous[†]
*Sinutab (Warner/Lambert): tablets	Phenylpropanolamine HCl, 25 mg	Phenyltoloxamine citrate, 22 mg	Acetaminophen, 325 mg	
*Sudafed (Burroughs Wellcome): tablets, syrup	Pseudoephedrine HCl, 30, 60 mg (tablets), 30 mg (syrup)	Chlorpheniramine maleate, 2 mg (syrup)		
Teldrin Multi-Symptom (Menley & James): capsules	Pseudoephedrine HCl, 30 mg	Chlorpheniramine maleate, 2 mg	Acetaminophen, 325 mg	
Triaminic Syrup (Dorsey): syrup	Phenylpropanolamine HCl, 12.5 mg	Chlorpheniramine maleate, 2 mg		
Triaminic Oral Infant Drops (Dorsey): drops	Phenylpropanolamine HCl, 20 mg/ml	Pheniramine maleate, 10 mg/ml pyrilamine maleate, 10 mg/ml		
Triaminic Tablets (Dorsey): tablets (timed-release)	Phenylpropanolamine HCl, 50 mg	Pheniramine maleate, 25 mg; pyrilamine maleate, 25 mg		

* Nonprescription.
† Milligrams in solid dosage form or 5 ml of liquid (except drops).

ANTIBIOTIC THERAPY OF INFECTIOUS DISEASES

Reproduced with permission from M. A. Sande and G. L. Mandell, "Antimicrobial Agents: General Considerations," in A. G. Gilman, L. S. Goodman, T. W. Rall, and F. Murad (eds.), *The Pharmacological Basis of Therapeutics,* 7th ed., Macmillan, New York, 1985, pp. 1072–1081.

Current use of antimicrobial agents in the therapy of infections

Presentation of choices of specific agents for the treatment of various infections is always provocative of discussion and disagreement because such choices often represent the distillate of personal experiences that may not duplicate those of others. In addition, the current availability of a number of drugs that are approximately equally effective makes an order of choice very difficult, if not impossible. To complicate matters, patterns of sensitivity of a number of microorganisms often vary with the hospital or clinic in which they are isolated; in some instances, this reflects a varying degree of exposure to specific agents. The material presented in this table represents not only the practice of the authors, based on their experience with the management of these infections, but also that of other experts in the United States. These drug selections represent initial therapy only. Each choice must be verified by testing of the etiological isolate for sensitivity to antibiotics. It is important to stress that, as more information accumulates, as recently introduced drugs are used for longer periods, and as entirely new agents are developed, some of the recommendations will require modification not only in the order of choice but even in the specific drugs that are suggested.

	Diseases	Drug order of choice		
		1st	2d[1]	3d[1]
I. Gram-positive cocci				
Staphylococcus aureus[*]	Penicillin G[2] sensitive — Abscesses, Bacteremia, Endocarditis, Pneumonia, Meningitis, Osteomyelitis, Cellulitis, Other	Penicillin G	A cephalosporin (G1)[3] Vancomycin	Clindamycin[4]
	Penicillin G resistant	A penicillinase-resistant penicillin	A cephalosporin (G1)[3] Vancomycin	
	Methicillin resistant	Vancomycin[5]	Trimethoprim-sulfamethoxazole + rifampin[6]	—
Streptococcus pyogenes	Pharyngitis, Scarlet fever, Otitis media, sinusitis, Cellulitis, Erysipelas, Pneumonia, Bacteremia, Other systemic infections	Penicillin G Penicillin V	A cephalosporin (G1)[3,7] Erythromycin	Vancomycin[7]

[*] All strains must be examined in *vitro* for sensitivity to various antimicrobial agents.
[1] Drugs included for second and third choices are (a) indicated in patients hypersensitive to equally or more effective agents, (b) potentially more dangerous than equally active drugs, (c) less likely to produce the desired therapeutic response, or (d) in need, in some cases, of further study in order to allow a valid evaluation of their efficacy.
[2] Minimal inhibitory concentration (MIC) is less than 0.2 µg/ml.
[3] G1 and G3 designate first- and third-generation cephalosporins, respectively. If no generation is specified, certain agents may be preferable to others. Therapeutic concentrations of most cephalosporins may not be achieved in the cerebrospinal fluid (exceptions include cefotaxime and moxalactam), and alternative agents should be used to treat infections of the CNS.
[4] Therapeutic concentrations are not achieved in the cerebrospinal fluid, and alternative agents should be used to treat infections of the CNS.
[5] Vancomycin is the only antimicrobial agent proven to be effective for treatment of serious infections due to methicillin-resistant S. aureus.
[6] Rifampin is highly active against most strains of S. aureus, including some that are resistant to methicillin. Since resistance develops rapidly (one-step mutation) during therapy, a second active drug, such as trimethoprim-sulfamethoxazole, should be used concurrently.
[7] Especially for bacteremia.

I. Gram-positive cocci (continued)	Diseases	Drug order of choice		
		1st	2d[1]	3d[1]
Streptococcus* (viridans group)	Endocarditis Bacteremia	Penicillin G ± streptomycin or gentamicin	A cephalosporin (G1)[3]	Vancomycin
Streptococcus agalactiae (group B)	Septicemia	Ampicillin or penicillin G ± an aminoglycoside	A cephalosporin (G1)[3]	Erythromycin
	Meningitis		Cefotaxime	Chloramphenicol[8]
Streptococcus faecalis* (enterococus)	Endocarditis	Penicillin G + gentamicin or streptomycin	Vancomycin + gentamicin or streptomycin	—
	Urinary tract infection	Ampicillin or penicillin G	Vancomycin	Nitrofurantoin
	Bacteremia			—
Streptococcus bovis	Endocarditis Urinary tract infection Bacteremia	Penicillin G ± streptomycin or gentamicin	A cephalosporin (G1)[3] ± streptomycin or gentamicin	Vancomycin
Streptococcus* (anaerobic species)	Bacteremia Endocarditis Brain and other abscesses Sinusitis	Penicillin G[9]	A cephalosporin (G1)[3] Clindamycin[4]	Chloramphenicol[8] Erythromycin[4]
Streptococcus pneumoniae* (pneumococcus)	Pneumonia Endocarditis Arthritis Sinusitis Otitis	Penicillin G	A cephalosporin (G1)[3] Erythromycin	Chloramphenicol Clindamycin
	Meningitis		Chloramphenicol[8] or cefotaxime	—

[8] Chloramphenicol is effective for infection of the CNS in patients who are allergic to betalactam antibiotics.
[9] Large doses of penicillin G may be required.

(continued)

Current use of antimicrobial agents in the therapy of infections *(continued)*

Diseases			Drug order of choice			
II. Gram-negative cocci			*1st*	*2d[1]*	*3d[1]*
Neisseria gonorrhoeae (gonococcus)	Genital infections	Penicillin sensitive	Ampicillin or amoxicillin Penicillin G A tetracycline	Erythromycin Spectinomycin	—
		Penicillinase producing	Spectinomycin	Cefoxitin or cefotaxime	Trimethoprim-sulfamethoxazole
	Arthritis-dermatitis syndrome		Ampicillin or amoxicillin Penicillin G	A tetracycline	Erythromycin
Neisseria meningitidis (meningococcus)	Meningitis Bacteremia		Penicillin G	Cefotaxime or moxalactan	Chloramphenicol[8]
	Carrier state		Rifampin	Minocycline	—

Diseases		*1st*	*2d[1]*	*3d[1]*
III. Gram-positive bacilli				
Bacillus anthracis*	"Malignant pustule" Pneumonia	Penicillin G	Erythromycin A tetracycline	A cephalosporin (G1)[3] Chloramphenicol
Corynebacterium diphtheriae[10]	Pharyngitis Laryngotracheitis Pneumonia Other local lesions	Penicillin G	Erythromycin	A cephalosporin (G1)[3] Rifampin
	Carrier state	Erythromycin	Penicillin G	—
Corynebacterium species, aerobic and anaerobic* (diphtheroids)	Endocarditis Infected foreign bodies	Penicillin G ± an aminoglycoside Vancomycin	Rifampin + penicillin G	—
Listeria monocytogenes	Meningitis Bacteremia Endocarditis	Ampicillin or penicillin G ± an aminoglycoside	Chloramphenicol[8] Erythromycin A tetracycline	—
Erysipelothrix rhusiopathiae	Erysipeloid	Penicillin G	Erythromycin A tetracycline	Chloramphenicol

[10] Antibiotics alone do not alter the clinical course of diphtheria, but drugs can eradicate the carrier state.

266

		Drug order of choice		
III. Gram-positive bacilli (continued)	*Diseases*	*1st*	*2d[1]*	*3d[1]*
*Clostridium perfringens** and other species	Gas gangrene[11]	Penicillin G	Chloramphenicol	A cephalosporin[3] Clindamycin
Clostridium tetani	Tetanus[11]	Penicillin G[12]	A tetracycline	Erythromycin
			Drug order of choice	
IV. Gram-negative bacilli	*Diseases*	*1st*	*2d[1]*	*3rd[1]*
*Escherichia coli**	Urinary tract infection[13]	Ampicillin ± an aminoglycoside A sulfonamide Trimethoprim-sulfamethoxazole	A cephalosporin[3] A tetracycline An aminoglycoside	Nitrofurantoin
	Other infections Bacteremia	Ampicillin ± an aminoglycoside	A cephalosporin[3] An aminoglycoside	Trimethoprim-sulfamethoxazole
*Enterobacter aerogenes**	Urinary tract[14] and other infections	Cefamandole, cefuroxime, or another cephalosporin (G3)[3] An aminoglycoside[15]	An antipseudomonal penicillin[16]	Trimethoprim-sulfamethoxazole
*Proteus mirabilis**	Urinary tract[14] and other infections	Ampicillin An aminoglycoside[15]	A cephalosporin[3]	—
*Proteus, other species**	Urinary tract[14] and other infections	An aminoglycoside[15] A cephalosporin (G3)[3]	An antipseudomonal penicillin[16]	—
*Pseudomonas aeruginosa**	Urinary tract infection[14]	An antipseudomonal penicillin[16]	An aminoglycoside[15]	—
	Pneumonia[17] Bacteremia[17]	An aminoglycoside[15] + antipseudomonal penicillin[16]	An aminoglycoside[15] + cefoperazone, ceftazidime, or cefsulodin[18]	—

11 Adequate debridement is absolutely essential.

12 Ten to 20 million units of penicillin G daily, with debridement and adsorbed tetanus toxoid.

13 Sulfonamides, trimethoprim-sulfamethoxazole, and urinary tract antiseptics are useful for acute urinary tract infections, especially cystitis, in the patient without obstructive uropathy or in whom the disease has not become chronic. These agents also prove useful for chronic suppressive therapy in patients with recurrent urinary tract infection. Some clinicians prefer to reserve the antibiotics, such as ampicillin and aminoglycosides, for cases in which there are systemic manifestations—particularly in acute pyelonephritis. In some areas, 20 to 40% of *E. coli* infections acquired in the community are resistant to ampicillin.

14 Urinary tract infections caused by microorganisms other than *E. coli* are less usual and frequently occur in the setting of obstructive uropathy or an indwelling urinary catheter, or following recurrent infections and the use of antibiotics. Therapy must be individualized but is frequently unsuccessful unless the underlying condition is corrected.

15 Gentamicin, tobramycin, amikacin, or netilmicin only.

16 Carbenicillin, ticarcillin, piperacillin, mezlocillin, or azlocillin.

17 While single-drug therapy with an antipseudomonal penicillin or an aminoglycoside is adequate for some infections caused by *P. aeruginosa*, the combination of the two classes of drug is recommended for therapy of serious infections, especially in the neutropenic patient or in the individual with pneumonia.

18 Cephalosporins that are most active against *P. aeruginosa* include cefoperazone, ceftazidime, and cefsulodin, but resistance may develop during therapy.

(continued)

Current use of antimicrobial agents in the therapy of infections (continued)

IV. Gram-negative baccilli (continued) Diseases	Drug order of choice		
	1st	2d[1]	3d[1]
Klebsiella pneumoniae*			
Urinary tract infection[14]	A cephalosporin[3]	An aminoglycoside Mezlocillin or piperacillin	Trimethoprim-sulfamethoxazole
Pneumonia	A cephalosporin[19] + an aminoglycoside	Mezlocillin or piperacillin ± an aminoglycoside	—
Salmonella*			
Typhoid fever Paratyphoid fever Bacteremia	Chloramphenicol Trimethoprim-sulfamethoxazole	Ampicillin[20]	Cefoperazone
Acute gastroenteritis	No therapy or trimethoprim-sulfamethoxazole	—	—
Shigella*			
Acute gastroenteritis	Trimethoprim-sulfamethoxazole	Ampicillin[20]	A tetracycline
Serratia*			
Variety of nosocomial and opportunistic infections	Gentamicin Cefoxitin or another cephalosporin (G3)[3]	Other aminoglycosides Antipseudomonal penicillins[16]	—
Acinetobacter*			
Various nosocomial infections	An aminoglycoside[15]	A cephalosporin (G3)[3]	—
Haemophilus influenzae*			
Otitis media Sinusitis Bronchitis	Amoxicillin or ampicillin[20] Trimethoprim-sulfamethoxazole	Cefaclor	—
Epiglottis Pneumonia Meningitis	Chloramphenicol Cefotaxime or moxalactam	Cefamandole[21] or cefuroxime[3] Ampicillin[20]	—
Haemophilus ducreyi			
Chancroid	Trimethoprim-sulfamethoxazole	A sulfonamide A tetracycline	Streptomycin
Brucella			
Brucellosis	A tetracycline ± streptomycin[22] or rifampin	Chloramphenicol ± streptomycin[22]	Trimethoprim-sulfamethoxazole
Yersinia pestis			
Plague	Streptomycin ± a tetracycline	A tetracycline	Chloramphenicol

[19] An increasing number of strains are becoming resistant to the first- and second-generation cephalosporins. Many authorities would use a cephalosporin with an aminoglycoside for treatment of pneumonia.
[20] Many strains are not now resistant to ampicillin or amoxicillin.
[21] Cefamandole should not be used for the therapy of *H. influenzae* meningitis.
[22] Such combined therapy is useful in severe infections.

| IV. Gram-negative bacilli (continued) | Diseases | Drug order of choice | | |
		1st	2d[1]	3d[1]
Yersinia enterocolitica	Yersiniosis	No treatment or trimethoprim-sulfamethoxazole[23]	—	—
	Sepsis	An aminoglycoside Chloramphenicol[24]		
Francisella tularensis	Tularemia	Streptomycin	A tetracycline	Chloramphenicol
Pasturella multocida	Wound infection (animal bites) Abscesses Bacteremia Meningitis	Penicillin G	A tetracycline[4] A cephalosporin (G1)[3]	—
Vibrio cholerae	Cholera	A tetracycline	Trimethoprim-sulfamethoxazole	Chloramphenicol
Falcobacterium meningosepticum	Meningitis	Erythromycin + rifampin	—	—
Pseudomonas mallei	Glanders	Streptomycin + a tetracycline	Streptomycin + chloramphenicol	—
Pseudomonas pseudomallei	Melioidosis	A tetracycline ± chloramphenicol	Chloramphenicol	Trimethoprim-sulfamethoxazole
Campylobacter jejuni	Enteritis	No treatment or erythromycin	A tetracycline Clindamycin	—
Campylobacter fetus*	Bacteremia	Chloramphenicol[24] Gentamicin	—	—
Bacteroides species (oral, pharyngeal)	Oral disease Sinusitis Brain abscess Lung abscess	Penicillin G[25] Clindamycin[4]	Metronidazole[25] Cefoxitin or moxalactam	Chloramphenicol[25] Erythromycin A tetracycline
Bacteroides fragilis	Brain abscess Lung abscess Intra-abdominal abscess Empyema Bacteremia Endocarditis	Clindamycin[4] Metronidazole[25,26]	Cefoxitin[4] or moxalactam[25]	Chloramphenicol[25] Piperacillin

[23] Data on treatment are sparse, but therapy with trimethoprim-sulfamethoxazole has been successful in some cases.
[24] Most strains are sensitive to aminoglycosides, but chloramphenicol is recommended in CNS infections.
[25] Preferred antibiotic for CNS infections.
[26] Metronidazole is bactericidal against B. fragilis and is thus recommended in endocarditis.

(continued)

Current use of antimicrobial agents in the therapy of infections (continued)

		Drug order of choice		
	Diseases	1st	2d[1]	3d[1]
IV. Gram-negative bacilli (continued)				
Fusobacterium nucleatum	Ulcerative pharyngitis, Lung abscess, empyema, Genital infections, Gingivitis	Penicillin G, Clindamycin	Cefoxitin, Metronidazole	Erythromycin, A tetracycline, Chloramphenicol
Calymmatobacterium granulomatis	Granuloma inguinale	A tetracycline	Streptomycin	—
Streptobacillus moniliformis	Bacteremia, Arthritis, Endocarditis, Abscesses	Penicillin G	Streptomycin, A tetracycline	—
Legionella pneumophila	Legionnaires' disease	Erythromycin ± rifampin	—	—
		Drug order of choice		
	Diseases	1st	2d[1]	3d[1]
V. Acid-fast bacilli				
Mycobacterium tuberculosis[27]	Pulmonary	Isoniazid + rifampin[28]	Isoniazid + ethambutol[28]	Rifampin + ethambutol
	Miliary, renal, meningeal, and other tuberculous infections	Isoniazid + rifampin, Isoniazid + rifampin + streptomycin[29] or ethambutol	—	—
Mycobacterium leprae	Leprosy	Dapsone + rifampin	Clofazimine	—
		Drug order of choice		
	Diseases	1st	2d[1]	3d[1]
VI. Spirochetes				
Treponema pallidum	Syphilis	Penicillin G	A tetracycline	Erythromycin
Treponema pertenue	Yaws	Penicillin G	A tetracycline	—
Borrelia recurrentis	Relapsing fever	A tetracycline	Penicillin G	—

27 Second- and third-choice drugs are available for the treatment of disease caused by M. tuberculosis.
28 Use isoniazid, ethambutol, and rifampin when primary resistance is likely.
29 Recommended by many clinicians for more severe forms of tuberculosis, such as meningitis and the disseminated (miliary) disease. Other physicians use only two of these agents, combining isoniazid and rifampin.

VI. Spirochetes (continued) Diseases		Drug order of choice		
		1st	*2d[1]*	*3d[1]*
Leptospira	Weil's disease Meningitis	Penicillin G	A tetracycline[4,30]	—
Lyme's disease agent	Lyme's disease	A tetracycline	Penicillin G	—

VII. Actinomycetes Diseases		Drug order of choice		
		1st	*2d[1]*	*3d[1]*
Actinomyces israelii	Cervicofacial, abdominal, thoracic, and other lesions	Penicillin G	A tetracycline	A cephalosporin[3] Chloramphenicol
Nocardia*	Pulmonary lesions Brain abscess Lesions of other organs	A sulfonamide ± ampicillin	A sulfonamide ± minocycline Trimethoprim-sulfamethoxazole[23]	—

VIII. Miscellaneous agents Diseases		Drug order of choice		
		1st	*2d[1]*	*3d[1]*
Ureaplasma urealyticum	Nonspecific urethritis	A tetracycline	Erythromycin	—
Mycoplasma pneumoniae	"Atypical pneumonia"	Erythromycin A tetracycline	—	—
Rickettsia	Typhus fever Murine typhus Brill's disease Rocky Mountain spotted fever Q fever Rickettsialpox	Chloramphenicol A tetracycline	—	—
Chlamydia psittaci	Psittacosis (ornithosis)	A tetracycline	Chloramphenicol	—

30 Some physicians favor a tetracycline over penicillin G as the drug of first choice.
31 A tetracycline may be given orally alone, or it may be applied locally in the conjunctival sac while a sulfonamide is being administered orally.

(continued)

Current use of antimicrobial agents in the therapy of infections (*continued*)

		Drug order of choice		
	Diseases	*1st*	*2d*[1]	*3d*[1]
VIII. Miscellaneous agents (continued)				
Chlamydia trachomatis	Lymphogranuloma venereum	A tetracycline	Erythromycin A sulfonamide	Chloramphenicol
	Trachoma	A sulfonamide + a tetracycline[31]	Erythromycin A tetracycline	Chloramphenicol
	Inclusion conjunctivitis (blennorrhea)	Erythromycin	—	—
	Nonspecific urethritis	A tetracycline	Erythromycin	A sulfonamide
Pneumocytis carinii	Pneumonia in impaired host	Trimethoprim-sulfamethoxazole	Pentamidine	—
		Drug order of choice		
	Diseases	*1st*	*2d*[1]	*3d*[1]
IX. Fungi				
Candida species	Skin and mucocutaneous lesions	Ketoconazole Nystatin[32] Clotrimazole[32]	Amphotericin B	—
	Urinary tract infection	Flucytosine[33] Amphotericin B[34]	—	—
	Disseminated disease	Amphotericin B	—	—
Coccidioides immitis	Pulmonary/pleural disease	No treatment or ketoconazole	Amphotericin B[35]	—
	Bone/joint or chronic pulmonary infection	Amphotericin B	Ketoconazole	—
	Meningeal disease	Amphotericin B[36]	—	—
Cryptococcus neoformans	Nonmeningeal disease	No treatment or amphotericin B ± flucytosine[37]		—
	Meningitis	Amphotericin B ± flucytosine[38]	—	—

32 Topical application.
33 A significant percentage of strains may be resistant or may become resistant during therapy.
34 As a bladder irrigant.
35 Low-dose treatment for patients disposed to dissemination.
36 Intrathecal and intravenous treatment with amphotericin B may be necessary.
37 For progressive disease or when there is evidence of dissemination.
38 The combination appears to give superior therapeutic results.

Drug order of choice

IX. Fungi (continued)

Diseases	1st	2d¹	3d¹
Histoplasma capsulatum			
Pulmonary disease	No treatment or ketoconazole	—	—
Disseminated disease	Amphotericin B[36]	Ketoconazole[4]	—
Aspergillus			
Invasive disease	Amphotericin B[36]	—	—
Mucor			
Invasive disease	Amphotericin B[36]	—	—
Blastomyces dermatitidis			
Blastomycosis (North American)	Amphotericin B	Ketoconazole	—
Sporothrix schenckii			
Sporotrichosis	Iodides	Amphotericin B	—

Drug order of choice

X. Viruses

Diseases	1st	2d¹	3d¹
Herpes simplex virus			
Genital disease	Acyclovir[39]	—	—
Keratoconjunctivitis	Vidarabine[40]	Idoxuridine[32]	—
Encephalitis	Vidarabine[40]	Acyclovir[40]	—
Influenza virus A			
Influenza	Amantadine[41] or rimantadine[41]	—	—

[39] Topical application or oral treatment.
[40] Parenteral.
[41] Effective as prophylaxis for Asian A_2 influenza virus. Some authorities recommend amantadine for treatment of established disease.

APPENDIX **IV**

PHARMACOLOGIC AGENTS USED IN TREATING CANCER

Reproduced with permission from P. Calabresi and R. E. Parks, Jr., "Chemotherapy of Neoplastic Diseases: Introduction," in A. G. Gilman, L. S. Goodman, T. W. Rall, and F. Murad (eds.), *The Pharmacological Basis of Therapeutics*, 7th ed., Macmillan, New York, 1985, pp. 1243–1245.

Drugs used to treat cancer

Class	Type of agent	Nonproprietary names (other names)	Disease
Alkylating agents	Nitrogen mustards	Mechlorethamine (HN₂)	Hodgkin's disease, non-Hodgkin's lymphomas
		Cyclophosphamide	Acute and chronic lymphocytic leukemias, Hodgkin's disease, non-Hodgkin's lymphomas, multiple myeloma, neuroblastoma, breast, ovary, lung, Wilms' tumor, rhabdomyosarcoma
		Melphalan (L-sarcolysin)	Multiple myeloma, breast, ovary
		Uracil mustard	Chronic lymphocytic leukemia, non-Hodgkin's lymphomas, Hodgkin's disease, ovary, primary thrombocytosis
		Chlorambucil	Chronic lymphocytic leukemia, primary macroglobulinemia, non-Hodgkin's lymphomas
	Alkyl sulfonates	Busulfan	Chronic granulocytic leukemia
	Nitrosoureas	Carmustine (BCNU)	Hodgkin's disease, non-Hodgkin's lymphomas, primary brain tumors, multiple myeloma, malignant melanoma
		Lomustine (CCNU)	Hodgkin's disease, non-Hodgkin's lymphomas, primary brain tumors, small-cell lung
		Semustine (methyl-CCNU)	Primary brain tumors, stomach, colon
		Streptozocin (streptozotocin	Malignant pancreatic insulinoma, malignant carcinoid
	Triazenes	Dacarbazine (DTIC; dimethyltriazenoimi-dazolecarboxamide)	Malignant melanoma, Hodgkin's disease, soft-tissue sarcomas
Antimetabolites	Folic acid analogs	Methotrexate (amethopterin)	Acute lymphocytic leukemia, choriocarcinoma, mycosis fungoides, breast, head and neck, lung, osteogenic sarcoma
	Pyrimidine analogs	Fluorouracil-(5-fluorouracil; 5-FU)	Breast, colon, stomach, pancreas, ovary, head and neck, urinary bladder, premalignant skin lesions (topical)
		Cytarabine (cytosine arabinoside)	Acute granulocytic and acute lymphocytic leukemias
	Purine analogs	Mercaptopurine (6-mercaptopurine; 6-MP)	Acute lymphocytic, acute granulocytic, and chronic granulocytic leukemias
		Thioguanine (6-thioguanine; TG)	Acute granulocytic, acute lymphocytic, and chronic granulocytic leukemias
Hormones and antagonists	Adrenocorticosteroids	Prednisone (several other equivalent preparations available)	Acute and chronic lymphocytic leukemias, non-Hodgkin's lymphomas, Hodgkin's disease, breast
	Progestins	Hydroxyprogesterone caproate Medroxyprogesterone acetate Megestrol acetate	Endometrium, breast

(continued)

Drugs used to treat cancer *(continued)*

Class	Type of agent	Nonproprietary names (other names)	Disease
Hormones and antagonists (continued)	Estogens	Diethylstilbestrol Ethinyl estradiol (other preparations available)	Breast, prostate
	Antiestrogen	Tamoxifen	Breast
	Androgens	Testosterone propionate Fluoxymesterone (other preparations available)	Breast
Natural products	Vinca alkaloids	Vinblastine (VLB)	Hodgkin's disease, non-Hodgkin's lymphomas, breast, testis
		Vincristine	Acute lymphocytic leukemia, neuroblastoma, Wilms' tumor, rhabdomyosarcoma, Hodgkin's disease, non-Hodgkin's lymphomas, small-cell lung
		Vindesine	Lymphomas, blastic crisis of chronic granulocytic leukemia, systemic mastocytosis
	Epidophyllotoxins	Etoposide Teniposide	Testis, small-cell lung and other lung, breast, Hodgkin's disease, non-Hodgkin's lymphomas, acute granulocytic leukemia, Kaposi's sarcoma
	Antibiotics	Dactinomycin (actinomycin D)	Choriocarcinoma, Wilms' tumor, rhabdomyosarcoma, testis, Kaposi's sarcoma
		Daunorubincin (daunomycin; rubidomycin)	Acute granulocytic and acute lymphocytic leukemias
		Doxorubicin	Soft-tissue, osteogenic, and other sarcomas; Hodgkin's disease, non-Hodgkin's lymphomas, acute leukemias, breast, genitourinary, thyroid, lung, stomach, neuroblastoma
		Bleomycin	Testis, head and neck, skin, esophagus, lung, genitourinary tract; Hodgkin's disease, non-Hodgkin's lymphomas
		Plicamycin (mithramycin)	Testis, malignant hypercalcemia
		Mitomycin (mitomycin C)	Stomach, cervix, colon, breast, pancreas, bladder, head and neck
	Enzymes	L-Asparaginase	Acute lymphocytic leukemia
Miscellaneous agents	Platinum coordination complexes	Cisplatin (*cis*-DDP)	Testis, ovary, bladder, head and neck, lung, thyroid, cervix, endometrium, neuroblastoma, osteogenic sarcoma
	Substituted urea	Hydroxyurea	Chronic granulocytic leukemia, polycythemia vera, essential thrombocytosis, malignant melanoma
	Methyl hydrazine derivative	Procarbazine (N-methyl-hydrazine, MIH)	Hodgkin's disease
	Adrenocortical suppressant	Mitotaine (*o,p'*-DDD)	Adrenal cortex
		Aminoglutethimide	Breast

Note: Not all drugs are discussed in Chapter 21.

LISTING OF POISON CONTROL CENTERS IN THE UNITED STATES

The nearest poison control or information center is equipped to provide the latest information on how to deal with a poisoning emergency. To make reasonably certain that the telephone number you call will reach the nearest, most authoritative center, use the journal *Emergency Medicine* which lists an updated list of major poison control centers in the United States each spring. This list is reproduced on the following pages.

Designated state or regional control centers and other centers with a 24-hour poison control staff are listed in **boldface type** and those that also are certified by the American Association of Poison Control Centers have an asterisk (*). In some states, large designated centers coexist with small satellite hospitals and centers that can give out limited poisoning information. These smaller centers are listed in lightface type. All centers in the state are grouped alphabetically by city or town. When calling one of the smaller centers, it is important to specify that you are calling about a poisoning emergency or that you desire certain poisoning information.

It is suggested that the telephone number of the poison control center nearest you be placed in close proximity to each telephone.

The following list is reproduced with permission from *Emergency Medicine*, April 30, 1986, pp. 115–124.

POISONING HOTLINES

ALABAMA
Alabama Poison Center*
809 University Blvd., E.
Tuscaloosa 35401
(800) 462-0800 (statewide)
(205) 345-0600

Birmingham
The Children's Hospital
of Alabama Poison Control
Center
1600 Seventh Ave., S. 35233
(800) 292-6678 (statewide)
(205) 933-4050 (local)
        939-9201 (local)
        939-9202 (local)

ALASKA
Anchorage
Anchorage Poison Center
Providence Hospital
P.O. Box 196604
3200 Providence Dr. 99519-0604
(907) 563-3393
(800) 478-3393

Fairbanks
Fairbanks Poison Control Center
Fairbanks Memorial Hospital
1650 Cowles St. 99701
(907) 456-7182

ARIZONA
**Arizona Regional Poison Control
System***
Tucson
(800) 362-0101

Phoenix
Central Arizona Regional Poison
Management Center
St. Luke's Hospital Medical
Center
1800 E. Van Buren St. 85006
(602) 253-3334

Tucson
Arizona Poison and Drug
Information Center*
University of Arizona
Arizona Health Sciences Center
85724
(800) 362-0101 (statewide)
(602) 626-6016 (Tucson)

ARKANSAS
**Statewide Poison Control Drug
Information Center**
University of Arkansas for
Medical Sciences
College of Pharmacy
4301 W. Markham St.
Little Rock 72205
(800) 482-8948 (statewide)
(501) 666-5532 (Pulaski County)

CALIFORNIA
Los Angeles
**Los Angeles County Medical
Association
Regional Poison Information
Center**
1925 Wilshire Blvd. 90057
(213) 484-5151 (public)
        644-2121 (MDs and
        hospitals)

Orange
**University of California Poison
Control Center**
Irvine Medical Center
101 City Drive S., Rte. 78 92668
(714) 634-5988

Sacramento
**UCDMC Regional Poison
Control Center***
2315 Stockton Blvd. 95817
(916)453-3692 (emergency poison
information)
(916) 453-3414 (nonemergency,
business information)

San Diego
**San Diego Regional Poison
Center***
University of California
San Diego Medical Center
225 Dickinson St. 92103
(619) 294-6000

San Francisco
**San Francisco Bay Area
Regional Poison Center***
San Francisco General Hospital
Room 1 E 86
1001 Potrero Ave. 94110
(415) 476-6600

San Jose
**Central-Coast Counties
Regional Poison Control Center**
Santa Clara Valley Medical
Center
751 S. Bascom Ave. 95128
(800) 662-9886
(408) 299-5112

Fresno
**Fresno Regional Poison Control
Center of Fresno Community
Hospital & Medical Center**
Fresno & R Sts. 93715
(209) 445-1222

Oakland
Children's Hospital Medical
Center of Northern California
747 52nd St. 94609
(415) 428-3248

COLORADO
Rocky Mountain Poison Center*
645 Bannock St.
Denver 80204-4507
(800) 332-3073
(303) 629-1123

CONNECTICUT
**Connecticut Poison Control
Center**

University of Connecticut
Health Center
Farmington 06032
(203) 674-3456
 674-3457

Bridgeport
St. Vincent's Medical Center
2800 Main St. 06606
(203) 576-5178

DELAWARE
Poison Information Center
Medical Center of Delaware
Wilmington Division
501 W. 14th St.
Wilmington 19899
(302) 655-3389

District of Columbia
National Capital Poison Center*
Georgetown University Hospital
3800 Reservoir Rd.
Washington 20007
(202) 625-3333

FLORIDA
Ft. Lauderdale
Broward General Medical Center
Poison Control Center
Emergency Department
1600 S. Andrews Ave. 33316
(305) 463-3131, ext. 1955, 1956

Jacksonville
St. Vincent's Medical Center
1800 Barrs St. 32203
(904) 387-7500
 387-7499 (TTY)

Tallahassee
Tallahassee Memorial Regional
Medical Center
1300 Miccosukee Rd. 32308
(904) 681-5411

Tampa
**Tampa Bay Regional Poison
Control Center***
Tampa General Hospital
Davis Island 33606
(800) 282-3171
(813) 251-6995

GEORGIA
Georgia Poison Control Center*
Grady Memorial Hospital
80 Butler St., S.E.
Atlanta 30335
(800) 282-5846
(404) 589-4400
    525-3323 (TTY)

Macon
Regional Poison Control Center
Medical Center of Central
Georgia
777 Hemlock St. 31201
(912) 744-1427
    744-1146
    744-1000

Savannah
Savannah Regional Poison
Control Center
Department of Emergency
Medicine
Memorial Medical Center 31403
(912) 355-5228

HAWAII
Hawaii Poison Center
Kapiolani-Children's Medical
Center
1319 Punahou St.
Honolulu 96826
(800) 362-3585
(808) 941-4411

IDAHO
Boise
**Idaho Emergency Medical
Poison Center***
St. Alphonsus Regional Medical
Center

1055 N. Curtis Rd. 83704
(800) 632-8000
(208) 334-2241

Pocatello
Idaho Drug Information Service
and Regional Poison Control
Center
Pocatello Regional Medical
Center
755 Hospital Way, Suite F-2
83201
(800) 632-9490 (Idaho only)
(208) 234-0777

ILLINOIS
**Chicago and Northeastern
Illinois
Regional Poison Control Center**
Rush-Presbyterian-St. Luke's
Medical Center
1753 W. Congress Pkwy.
Chicago 60612
(800) 942-5969 (Illinois only)
(312) 942-5969

Peoria Poison Center
St. Francis Hospital Medical
Center
530 N.E. Glen Oak Ave.
Peoria 61637
(800) 322-5330
(309) 672-2334

**Central and Southern Illinois
Regional Poison Resource
Center***
St. Johns's Hospital
800 E. Carpenter St.
Springfield 62769
(800) 252-2022
(217) 753-3330

INDIANA
Indiana Poison Center*
1001 W. 10th St.
Indianapolis 46202
(800) 382-9097 (Indiana only)
(317) 630-7351

Blue Ridge
Parkview Memorial Hospital
2200 Randalia Dr.
Ft. Wayne 46805
(219) 484-6636

IOWA
University of Iowa Hospitals and Clinics
Poison Control Center*
Iowa City 52242
(800) 272-6477
(319) 356-2922

Des Moines
Variety Club Poison and Drug Information Center
Iowa Methodist Medical Center
1200 Pleasant St. 50308
(800) 362-2327
(515) 283-6254

KANSAS
Mid-America Poison Center
University of Kansas Medical Center
39th & Rainbow Blvd.
Kansas City 66103
(800) 332-6633
(913) 588-6633

Mid-Plains Poison Control Center*
Omaha, Neb.
(800) 228-9515

Wichita
Wesley Medical Center
550 N. Hillside Ave. 67214
(316) 688-2277

KENTUCKY
Ft. Thomas
St. Luke Hospital of Campbell County
Northern Kentucky Poison Center
85 N. Grand Ave. 41075

(800) 352-9900
(606) 572-3215

Louisville
Kentucky Regional Poison Center of Kosair Children's Hospital*
P.O. Box 35070 40232-5070
(800) 722-5725 (toll free in Kentucky)
(502) 589-8222 (metropolitan Louisville)

LOUISIANA
Louisiana Regional Poison Control Center*
1501 Kings Hwy
Shreveport 71130
(800) 535-0525
(318) 425-1524

MAINE
Maine Poison Control Center at Maine Medical Center
22 Bramhall St.
Portland 04102
(800) 442-6305
(207) 871-2381 (ER)

MARYLAND
Maryland Poison Center*
University of Maryland
School of Pharmacy
20 N. Pine St.
Baltimore 21201
(800) 492-2414 (Maryland only)
(301) 528-7701

MASSACHUSETTS
Massachusetts Poison Control System
300 Longwood Ave.
Boston 02115
(800) 682-9211
(617) 232-2120
277-3323 (TTY)

MICHIGAN
Poison Control Center*
Children's Hospital of Michigan
3901 Beaubien
Detroit 48201
(800) 572-1655 (rest of Michigan)
(800) 462-6642 (outside of metro
area 313)
(313) 745-5711

**Blodgett Regional Poison
Center***
Blodgett Memorial Medical
Center
1840 Wealthy St., S.E.
Grand Rapids 49506
(800) 632-2727
(616) 774-7854

Kalamazoo
Great Lakes Poison Center
Bronson Methodist Hospital
252 E. Lovell St. 49001
(800) 442-4112 (only in area code
616)
(616) 383-6409

MINNESOTA
Hennepin Poison Center*
Hennepin County Medical
Center
701 Park Ave.
Minneapolis 55415
(612) 347-3141

**Minnesota Poison Control
System***
St. Paul–Ramsey Medical Center
640 Jackson St.
St. Paul 55101
(800) 222-1222
(612) 221-2113

MISSISSIPPI
Regional Poison Control Center
University Medical Center
2500 N. State St.
Jackson 39216
(601) 354-7660

MISSOURI
**Cardinal Glennon Children's
Hospital
Regional Poison Center***
1465 S. Grand Blvd.
St. Louis 63104
(800) 392-9111
(314) 772-5200

Kansas City
The Children's Mercy Hospital
24th and Gillham Rd. 64108
(816) 234-3000

MONTANA
Rocky Mountain Poison Center*
Denver, Colo.
(800) 525-5042

NEBRASKA
**Mid-Plains Poison Control
Center***
Children's Memorial Hospital
8301 Dodge St.
Omaha 68114
(800) 642-9999 (outside Omaha)
(402) 390-5400 (Omaha)
(800) 228-9515 (Idaho, Iowa,
Kan., Mo., S.Dak.)

NEVADA
Las Vegas
Southern Nevada Memorial
Hospital
1800 W. Charleston Blvd. 89102
(702) 385-1277

NEW HAMPSHIRE
**New Hampshire Poison
Information Center**
2 Maynard St.
Hanover 03756
(800) 562-8236 (New Hampshire)
(603) 646-5000 (outside New
Hampshire)

NEW JERSEY
**New Jersey Poison Information
and Education System***

Newark Beth Israel Medical
Center
201 Lyons Ave
Newark 07112
(800) 962-1253
(201) 926-8005

NEW MEXICO
**New Mexico Poison and Drug
Information Center***
University of New Mexico
Albuquerque 87131
(800) 432-6866
(505) 843-2551
(505) 277-4261 (administration
only)

NEW YORK
Binghamton
Southern Tier Poison Center
Binghamton General Hospital
Mitchell Ave. 13903
(607) 723-8929

Buffalo
**Western New York Poison
Control Center at Children's
Hospital of Buffalo**
219 Bryant St. 14222
(716) 878-7654
      878-7655

East Meadow
**Long Island Regional Poison
Control Center***
Nassau County Medical Center
2201 Hempstead Tnpk. 11554
(516) 542-2324
      542-2325
      542-2323 (TTY)

New York
New York City Poison Center*
455 First Ave. 10016
(212) 340-4494
      764-7667

Nyack
Hudson Valley Poison Center

Nyack Hospital
N. Midland Ave. 10960
(914) 353-1000

Rochester
Finger Lakes Poison Center
LIFE LINE
University of Rochester
Medical Center
Box 777 14642
(716) 275-5151
      275-2700 (TTY)

Schenectady
Ellis Hospital Poison Center
1101 Nott St. 12308
(518) 382-4039
      382-4309

Syracuse
**Central New York Poison
Control Center**
Upstate Medical Center
750 E. Adams St. 13210
(315) 476-4766
(800) 252-5655 (outside
Onandaga County)

NORTH CAROLINA
Duke Poison Control Center*
Duke University Medical Center
Durham 27710
(800) 672-1697
(919) 684-8111

Asheville
Western NC Poison Control
Center
Memorial Mission Hospital
509 Biltmore Ave. 28801
(704) 255-4490

Charlotte
Mercy Hospital
2001 Vail Ave. 28207
(704) 379-5827

Greensboro
The Moses H. Cone Memorial
Hospital
Triad Poison Center
1200 N. Elm St. 27401-1020
(800) 722-2222 (North Carolina)
(919) 379-4105

Hickory
Catawba Memorial Hospital
Fairgrove Church Rd. 28601
(704) 322-6649

NORTH DAKOTA
North Dakota Poison Information
Center
St. Luke's Hospitals
Fifth St. N. & Mills Ave.
Fargo 58122
(800) 732-2200 (North Dakota
only)
         280-5575

OHIO
Central Ohio Poison Control
Center*
Children's Hospital
700 Children's Dr.
Columbus 43205
(800) 682-7625
(614) 228-1323

Southwest Ohio Regional Poison
Control System and Drug and
Poison Information Center*
University of Cincinnati Medical
Center
Medical Science Bldg. M.L. 144
231 Bethesda Ave.
Cincinnati 45267-0144
(800) 872-5111
(513) 872-5111

Akron
Akron Regional Poison Control
Center
Children's Hospital Medical
Center of Akron

281 Locust St. 44308
(800) 362-9922
(216) 379-8562

Cleveland
Greater Cleveland Poison
Control Center
2101 Adelbert Rd. 44106
(216) 231-4455

Dayton
Children's Medical Center
1 Children's Plaza 45404
(800) 762-0727
(513) 222-2227

Lorain
Lorain Community Hospital
3700 Kolbe Rd. 44053
(216) 282-2220
(800) 821-8972

Mansfield
Mansfield General Hospital
335 Glessner Ave. 44903
(419) 526-8200

Toledo
Poison Information Center
Medical College of Ohio
Hospital
3000 Arlington Ave. 43614
(419) 381-3897

Youngstown
Mahoning Valley Poison Center
St. Elizabeth Hospital Medical
Center
1044 Belmont Ave. 44501
(216) 746-2222
         746-5510 (TTY)

OKLAHOMA
Oklahoma Poison Control Center
Oklahoma Children's Memorial
Hospital
P.O. Box 26307
940 N.E. 10th 73126

Oklahoma City 73126
(800) 522-4611 (in state)
(405) 271-5454

OREGON
**Oregon Poison Control and Drug
Information Center**
University of Oregon Health
Sciences Center
3181 S. W. Sam Jackson Park Rd.
Portland 97201
(800) 452-7165
(503) 225-8968

PENNSYLVANIA
Allentown
Lehigh Valley Poison Center
Allentown Hospital
17th & Chew Sts. 18102
(215) 433-2311

Altoona
Keystone Region Poison Center
Mercy Hospital
2500 Seventh Ave. 16603
(814) 946-3711

Danville
Susquehanna Poison Center
Geisinger Medical Center
N. Academy Ave. 17821
(717) 271-6116

Erie
**Northwest Regional Poison
Center**
Saint Vincent Health Center
232 W. 25th St. 16544
(814) 452-3232

Hershey
Capital Area Poison Center
University Hospital
Milton S. Hershey Medical
Center
University Dr. 17033
(717) 534-6111
      534-6039

Jersey Shore
Jersey Shore Hospital
Thompson St. 17740
(717) 398-0100, ext. 225

Johnstown
Conemaugh Valley
Memorial Hospital
1086 Franklin St. 15905
(814) 535-5351

Philadelphia
**Delaware Valley Regional
Poison Control Center**
One Children's Center
34th & Civic Center Blvd. 19104
(215) 386-2066 (administration)
(215) 386-2100 (emergency)

Pittsburgh
Pittsburgh Poison Center*
Children's Hospital
One Children's Place
3705 Fifth Ave. at DeSoto St.
15213
(412) 681-6669 (emergency)
      647-5600 (admin./
      consultation)

RHODE ISLAND
**Rhode Island Poison Control
Center**
Rhode Island Hospital
593 Eddy St.
Providence 02902
(401) 277-5906

SOUTH CAROLINA
Palmetto Poison Center
University of South Carolina
College of Pharmacy
Columbia 29208
(800) 922-1117
(803) 765-7359

SOUTH DAKOTA
Mid-Plains Poison Control
Center*
Omaha, Neb.
(800) 228-9515

Aberdeen
Dakota Midland Poison Control
Center 57401
(605) 225-1880
(800) 592-1889

Rapid City
Rapid City Regional Poison
Center
353 Fairmont Blvd. 57701
(800) 742-8925
(605) 341-8222

Sioux Falls
McKennen Hospital Poison
Center
P.O. Box 5045
800 E. 21st St. 57117-5045
(800) 952-0123
        843-0505
(605) 336-3894

TENNESSEE
Chattanooga
T.C. Thompson Children's
Hospital
910 Blackford St. 37403
(615) 778-6100

Knoxville
Memorial Research Center and
Hospital
1924 Alcoa Hwy. 37920
(615) 544-9400

Memphis
Southern Poison Center, Inc.
848 Adams Ave. 38103
(901) 528-6048

TEXAS
Texas State Poison Center

University of Texas Medical
Branch
Eighth & Mechanic Sts.
Galveston 77550
(800) 392-8548 (Galveston)
(409) 765-1420 (Houston)
(512) 478-4490 (Austin)

Dallas
North Central Texas Poison
Center
P.O. Box 35926 75235
(800) 441-0040
(214) 920-2400

El Paso
El Paso Poison Control Center
R.E. Thomason General Hospital
4815 Alameda Ave. 79905
(915) 533-1244

UTAH
Intermountain Regional Poison
Control Center*
50 N. Medical Dr.
Salt Lake City 84132
(800) 662-0062
(801) 581-2151

VERMONT
Vermont Poison Center
Medical Center Hospital of
Vermont
Colchester Ave.
Burlington 05401
(802) 658-3456 (poison
information)
(802) 656-2721 (education
programs)

VIRGINIA
Charlottesville
Blue Ridge Poison Center
University of Virginia Hospital
22908
(800) 552-3723 (TTY: Va. only)
(800) 446-9876 (TTY)
(804) 924-5543

Norfolk
Tidewater Poison Center
150 Kingsley Lane 23505
(800) 552-6337
(804) 489-5288

Richomond
Central Virginia Poison Center
Medical College of Virginia
23298
(804) 786-4780 (business)
(804) 786-9123 (24-hour
emergency service)

Roanoke
Southwest Virginia Poison
Center
Roanoke Memorial Hospitals
P.O. Box 13367
Belleview at Jefferson St. 24033
(703) 981-7336

WASHINGTON
Seattle
Seattle Poison Center*
Children's Orthopedic Hospital
and Medical Center
4800 Sand Point Way, N.E.
P.O. Box C5371 98105-9990
(800) 732-6985 (statewide)
(206) 526-2121

Spokane
Spokane Poison Center
Deaconess Medical Center
800 W. Fifth Ave. 99210
(800) 572-5842 (statewide)
        541-5624 (N. Idaho and W.
        Montana)
(509) 747-1077 (TTY)

Tacoma
Mary Bridge Poison Center
Mary Bridge Children's Health
Center
P.O. Box 5588
311 S. L St. 98405
(800) 542-6319 (statewide)
(206) 594-1414

Yakima
**Central Washington Poison
Center**
Yakima Valley Memorial
Hospital
2811 Tieton Dr. 98902
(800) 572-9176 (statewide)
(509) 248-4400

WEST VIRGINIA
West Virginia Poison Center
West Virginia University
School of Pharmacy
3110 McCorkle Ave., S.E.
Charleston, W.V. 25304
(800) 642-3625
(304) 348-4211

WISCONSIN
Green Bay
**Green Bay Poison Control
Center**
St. Vincent Hospital
835 S. Van Buren St. 54305
(414) 433-8100

Madison
Madison Area Poison Center
University Hospital and Clinics
600 Highland Ave. 53792
(608) 262-3702

Milwaukee
Milwaukee Poison Center
Children's Hospital of Wisconsin
1700 W. Wisconsin AVe. 53233
(414) 931-4114

WYOMING
Wyoming Poison Center
DePaul Hospital
2600 E. 18th St.
Cheyenne 82001
(307) 777-7955

Rocky Mountain Poison Center*
Denver (800) 442-2702

DRUG INDEX

Parentheses indicate the page on which a structural formula appears.

enalapril (Vasotec), 87
ephedrine, (13), 14, 18, 107, 116
epinephrine (Adrenalin, Sus-phrine), (13), 15, 16, 114, 116, 118
ergonovine (Ergotrate), 40–(41), 166
ergotamine (Gynergen), 40
erythrityl tetranitrate (Cardilate), (77), 79, 80
erythromycin estolate (Ilosone), 202
erythromycin ethylsuccinate (E.E.S., Pediamycin), 202
erythromycin stearate (Ethril), 202
ethacrynic acid (Edecrin), 84, 85, (102), 104–105
ethambutol (Myambutol), 208–209

flavoxate (Urispas), 107, (108)
Fleet phospho soda, 121
fludrocortisone (Florinef), 137
fluorouracil (5-FU), 220
fluprednisolone (Alphadrol), 137
furosemide (Lasix), 84, 85, (102), 104–105

gallamine (Flaxedil), 31
gentamicin (Garamycin), 200
glipizide (Glucotrol), 147–149
glutethimide (Doriden), 245
glyburide (Diabeta, Micronase), 147–149
glycerin suppositories, 121, 127
glyceryl guaiacolate (Robitussin) 116
glycopyrrolate (Robinul), 33, 124
griseofulvin (Fulvicin, Grifulvin, Grisactin), 205
growth hormone (Protopin), 162–164
guanethidine (Ismelin), 20, 21

heparin, 93–95
hexamethonium, 28
human growth hormone (Protropin), 163
hydralazine (Apresoline), 84, 85–86, 89, 90
hydrochlorothiazide (Hydrodiuril, Esidrex), 84, (102), 104
hydroflumethiazide (Saluron), 104
hydroxychloroquine (Plaquenil), 211
hydroxyurea (Hydrea), 222

ibuprofen (Motrin), 43
idoxuridine (Herplex, Stoxil), 205–206
imipramine (Tofranil), 14, 18, 107, (108)
indomethacin (Indocin), 43, 93, 96
insulin, 142–147
iodine, 155–157
iodoquinol (Diodoquin), 210
ipecac, 243–244
isoetharine (in Bronkosol, Bronkometer), 14, 18, 116, 118

isoniazid (INH), 182, 208
isoproterenol (Isuprel, Medihaler-Iso), (13), 15, 17, 116, 118
isosorbide dinitrate (Isordil, Sorbitrate), 79, 80

kanamycin (Kantrex), 200
kaolin (Donnagel), 128

labetalol (Normodyne, Trandate), 19, 20, 79, 80, 89, 128
L-asparaginase, 222
lidocaine (Xylocaine), 69, 70, 71, 72, 73
lincomycin (Lincocin), 202–203
lomustine (CCNU), 217
loperamide (Imodium), 122, 128
LSD, 40, (41)
lypressin, 165–166

magnesium citrate, 121
magnesium hydroxide (Milk of Magnesia), 121, 126
magnesium sulfate, 167
malathion, (27)
mannitol, (103), 106
mebendazole (Vermox), 212
mechlorethamine (Mustargen), 217
meclizine (Antivert, Bonine), 37
melphalan (Alkeran), 217
mephentermine (Wyamine), 14, 18
mercaptopurine (Purinethol), (218)–219
metalazone (Zaroxolyn), 104
metaproterenol (Alupent, Metaprel), 14, 18, 116–(117), 118
metaraminol (Aramine), 14, 18
methapyrilene (Histadil), (38)
methenamine (Mandelamine), 194
methicillin (Staphcillin), 195–197
methimazole (Tapazole), (156)–157
methotrexate (Folex, Mexate), 218–(219)
methoxamine (Vasoxyl), 14, 18
methyclothiazide (Enduron, Aquatensin), 104
methyldopa (Aldomet), 19, 20, 88–89
methylergonovine (Methergine), 40, 166
methylprednisolone (Medrol), 137
methyltyrosine (Demser), 20, 21
methysergide (Sansert), 40, (41)
metoclopramide (Reglan), 121, 122–(123)
metocurine (Metubine), 31
metoprolol (Lopressor), 19, 20, 79, 80, 88
metronidazole (Flagyl), 210–211
mezlocillin (Mezlin), 195–197

succinylcholine (Anectine), 31, (32)
sulfasalazine (Azulfidine), 194
sulfisoxazole (Gantrisin), 194
sulfomethoxazole (Bactrim, Septra),
    193–194
sulfoxone (Diasone), 209

tabun, 28
tamoxifen (Nolvadex), 221
terbutaline (Brethine, Bricanyl), 14,
    18, 116–(117), 118
terfenadine (Seldane), 37, (39)
tetracycline, 200–201, 211
tetrahydrazoline (Tyzine), 114
theophylline (Slo-phylin, Theo-Dur),
    (117), 118
thiabendazole (Mintezol), 212
thiiodothyronine (Cytomel), 154
thioguanine, 219
thyroglobulin (Proloid), 154
thyroid, 150–157
thyroxine (Levothyroid, Synthroid),
    154
ticarcillin (Ticar), 195–197
timolol (Timoptic), 19, 20, 79
tincture of opium (Paregoric), 122,
    128
tobramycin (Nebcin), 200
tolazamide (Tolinase), 147–149
tolazoline (Priscoline), 19, 20
tolbutamide (Orinase), 147–149
tolnaftate (Tinactin), 204–205

triamcinolone (Kenalog, Aristocort),
    137
triamterene (Dyrenium), 84, 85, (103),
    105–106
trichlormethiazide (Naqua,
    Metahydrin), 104
trimethaphan (Arfonad), 28, 88
trimethoprim (Bactrim, Septra),
    193–194, 212
tripelennamine (Pyribenzamine), 37,
    (38)
triprolidine (Actidil), 37

undecylenic acid (Desenex), 204

vancomycin (Vancocin), 199, 204
vasopressin injection (Pitressin),
    165–166
verapamil (Calan), 68, 69, 71, 72,
    74–75, (77), 79, 81
vercuronium (Norcuron), 31
vidarabine (Vira-A), 206, 219
vinblastine (Velban), 222
vincristine (Oncovin), 222

warfarin (Coumadin), 93–96,
    175–176, 246–247

xylometazoline (Neosynephrine 2,
    Otrivin, Sinutab Long Lasting
    Nasal Spray), 114

GENERAL INDEX

Parentheses indicate the page on which a structural formula appears.

heart *continued*
  failure, 58–65, 89, 101, 134
  arrhythmias, 47–48, 52–55, 66–75
  valves, 47–48, 49–52
  block, 55
  coronary insufficiency, 76–82
Henle, loop of, 85, 100, 104–105
histamine, 34–40, (35)
  and drugs, 36–40
Hodgkin's disease, 217, 222
hormones
  adrenal, 133–141; *see also* steroids
  and cancer therapy, 221
  thyroid: *see* thyroid hormone
hydrochloric acid, 36, 39–40
hypertension, 19, 21, 43, 50–51,
    58–59, 78, 83–91, 101, 124, 134
hyperthyroidism, 154–156
hypoglycemic agents, 147–149; *see
  also individual agents*
hypothalamus, 135, 151–152, 161–165
hysterectomy and osteoporosis,
    159–160

immunity
  active, 233, 234–236
  passive, 233, 236–237
immunization schedule, 234–235
immunosuppressants, 227–232
immunotoxins, 231–232
inflamation
  and prostaglandins, 43
  and glucocorticoids, 138
insecticides, 27
  antidotes to, 246
insulin, 136, 142–147, 162
insufficiency, valvular, 52
iodide and iodine, 152–157

ketoacidosis, 143
kidneys
  physiology, 99–100
  drug effects on, 101–110
  and stone production, 109

labor
  induction of, 42
laxatives, 125–127
Legionnaire's disease, 201, 202
leprosy, 207, 209–210
Lugol's solution, 155
lymphocytes, 228–229, 231

malaria, 211–212
mannitol, (103), 106
mast cells, 35, 118
miniheparinization, 95
migraine, 40
mineralocorticoids, 133–135
mountain sickness, 106–107

multiple sclerosis, 140
myasthenia gravis, 26–27
myxedema, 151, 154

narcotics
  and cough, 115–116
  and diarrhea, 122, 127–128
neuromuscular transmission
  and drugs, 26, 28–33
  and thiamine, 178–179
niacin, 178–179, 181
nicotine and cigarettes, 23, 68, 78, 84
nicotine acid: *see* niacin
nitrogen mustards, 216–217
nitrosoureas, 217
norepinephrine, 12–21

obesity
  and thyroid hormone, 154
organ transplantation, 229–231
osmotic diuretics, 106; *see also*
    mannitol
osteomyelitis and clindamycin, 203
osteoporosis, 158, 159–160, 173–174
oxytocin, 162, 166

pacemakers, cardiac, 68
pancrease, 142–144
pantothenic acid, 184–185
para-amino-bonzoic acid, 191
parathyroid hormone, 157–158, 159
Parkinson's disease, 30
penicillinase, 193, 195–197, 204
penicillins, 195–197
peptic ulcer
  and atropine, 30
  and histamine, 36, 39–40
  treatment of, 121–125
pernicious anemia, 182–183
pheochromocytoma, 21
phenothiazines, 164
pituitary gland, 135, 151–152,
    161–167
plasma, fresh, 95–96
plasmapheresis, 27
platelets, 92–94, 96
  and amrinone, 65
  and glucocorticoids, 139
poison control centers, 242–243,
    277–287
poisoning, 241–147
  atropine, 26, 30
  treatment of, 242–247
polypeptide antibiotics, 204
potassium
  and digoxin, 64
  and diuretics, 104–106
pregnancy and iodine, 156
  and oxytocin, 166
  and tetracycline, 201

---

prolactin, 164
prostaglandins, (42)–43, 138, 166
prothrombin time, 95
protozoal infections, 210–212
pteroylglutamic acid; see folic acid
purine antagonists, 215, 219–220
pyridoxine, 178–179, 181–182
pyrimidine antagonists, 215, 220

receptors
  autonomic, 9–10
  adrenergic, 12–21
  cholinergic, 22–23
recombinant DNA, 144, 146, 163
renin, 87
respiratory system
  physiology, 111–113
  and drugs, 114–119
retrolental fibroplasia, 175
riboflavin, 178–181
rickets, 173–174

SA-node, 52–54, 66–68, 71–75
scurvy, 177
serotonin, 40–42, (41)
steroids, 115, 119
sexual dysfunction
  and drugs, 88–89
sick sinus syndrome, 68
stenosis, valvular, 52
steroids, 177; see also glucocorticoids
steroids and tumors, 221–222
stones, kidney, 177–178
sulfonamides, 193–195
systemic lupus erythematosus (SLE),
  139–140

tetracyclines, 200–201
thiamine, 178–180

thiazenes, 217
thiazide diuretics, 103–104
thrombin, 93–96
thyroid gland, 68
thyroid hormone, 150–154, 162
thyroxine, 150–153
toxoids, 233–235
tricyclic antidepressants
  and urinary incontinence, 107
triiodothyronine, 150–(153)
tuberculosis, 207–209, 228, 234–235

universal antidote, 245
urinary tract infection, 194–195
urologic disorders, 107–109
uterus, 40, 166–167

vaccines, 233–236
vasopressin, 102, 165–166
vitamin A, 171–173
vitamin B_1: see thiamine
vitamin B_2: see riboflavin
vitamin B_3: see niacin
vitamin B_5: see pantothenic acid
vitamin B_6: see pyridoxine
vitamin B_{12}: see cyanocobalamine
vitamin C, (176)–178
vitamin D, 157–160, 173–174
vitamin E, 174–175
vitamin K
  and coagulation, 93–96, 175–176
vitamin requirements, 170–171; see
  also individual agents
vitamins, 169–185; see also vitamin
  K; vitamin D

withdrawal, narcotic
  clonidine in, 19